Praise

MW00846751

"In the span of getting to know Dr. Gary Sprouse and reading his book, I have been introduced to many new concepts and ideas. His ideas and models for stress reduction are life-changing. You will absolutely love this. A must-read."

> —Jack Canfield, coauthor of *Chicken Soup for the Soul* and author of *The Success Principles*

"Dr. Sprouse, I was crouched in the corner of my bedroom with a phone and knife, trying to decide which one to use. I could envision the blood spurting from my neck, draining all the stress from my body. You were my best hope. I summoned all the strength I had left and called you. You didn't give me a lecture or a pep talk or get hysterical. You gave me three things I needed: empathy, caring, and a reason to live. I'm still alive this morning because of you and what you taught me about handling stress."

> —A Former Patient

"Dr. Sprouse, the 30 minutes I spent with you was more helpful than the 2 years I spent in counseling."

> —Robert P., a patient

"After filling out your worry sheet, I felt like a 200-pound weight was lifted off my shoulders."

> —Sharon C, Nurse Practitioner

"Dr. Sprouse, you gave me some self-esteem when I had none. You gave me hope when I had none. Dr. Sprouse, you gave me explanations that made sense when everything else was crazy. I'm so glad I met you. I don't think I would be here if it weren't for you. Thank you."

> —Betsy H., a patient

"I would highly recommend buying this book to anyone who wants to alleviate their chronic stress. By learning the root cause, I have been able to reduce my stress. One technique I learned was compartmentalization. My mind is clearer and now I can break down my stresses in a way that allows me to handle my anxieties and fears better."

—Cindy, a patient

"This book has changed my life in such a positive way! It has given me easy and practical tools to manage my anxieties, worries, and stress. One of my favorite parts is the Worry Organizer. By objectively looking at the facts around my worries, it has allowed me to worry less."

—Kim, a seminar attendee

"My sessions with Dr. Sprouse have been a breath of fresh air. He inspires me exponentially more than any of my previous treatments. I highly recommend Dr. Gary J. Sprouse as a result of my tremendous progress under his care."

—Gus, a patient

"I loved the book. What it did for me, even before I finished reading it, blew my mind. It began to change a pattern of stress I could not let go of for years. The greater the knowledge, the greater the change. This book is a must-read!"

—Susan, a patient

"The Highway to **My** Happy Place, Off we go! If you make someone better off because of an interaction with them, you have accomplished a lot. **This book is an easy read!**"

—Anny, a patient

"This book is filled with innovative strategies on how to reduce your daily stress level and how to regularly find your 'happy place,' something that eludes most of us. This book will be particularly helpful for those struggling to identify why they don't feel good and how to make the quality of their lives better. I highly recommend it!"

—Jennifer L. FitzPatrick, MSW, LCSW-C, CSP, Author of *Reimagining Customer Service in Healthcare* and *Cruising Through Caregiving*

"I have known Dr. Gary Sprouse since I was a young woman suffering from PTSD and a severe panic disorder. My struggles with stress led me down a dark path of self destruction and hopeless nihilism. Dr. Sprouse helped me to rearrange my perspective on many things, in a way I had never encountered. Stress being the biggest one, the root cause of my suffering. I am a tough nut to crack—but he managed to help me restore order to the chaotic mess that was my life. Dr. Sprouse gave me the tools to change my mindset, and that allowed me to apply coping mechanisms that I never knew existed. The process was cathartic and allowed me to know peace in a way I hadn't since childhood. I tremble to think where—or even if—I'd be, had I not had the great fortune of knowing him. I am forever changed and forever grateful to this man. He accomplished in me what countless therapists, psychologists, and counselors could not."

—Kelly G., seminar attendee

HIGHWAY TO YOUR
Happy Place

THE LESS STRESS DOC
GARY SPROUSE M.D.

HIGHWAY TO YOUR
Happy Place

A ROADMAP TO
LESS STRESS

Dedication

The roadmap to get a published book has stretched out over 25 years. That makes for a lot of people to thank.

I want to acknowledge Arthur Schwartz, a colleague of mine. We were both trying to get our books published 25 years ago. For 2 years we worked together to find an agent and a publisher. I realize now I was nowhere near ready then, but I did learn a lot during that time.

I want to thank Melissa Sherwood. We have been friends for 30 years. We have done a radio show and TV show together. We have been working on our book projects together over the years. She has been a beacon of hope and optimism that we would both become published authors someday.

I want to thank my first editor, Suzi Peel. I didn't always like the changes she made but she did make me rethink my terminology and the changes that came about from her constructive criticism led me to this finished project.

I am indebted to my first editor, and want to thank my second editor, Mary Dempsey. She was more helpful to me but she came in at a point of the book when I had a better idea of what I wanted to accomplish. She was able to ask questions that needed to be answered so that the book would be clear to every reader.

I want to thank Steve Harrison, his wife Laura, my coach Sarah Brown and Steve's team at Bradley Communications. For a wannabe author they were great teachers and mentors. Their programs helped me learn all that it takes to be an author and my readers are the benefactors of their skill and knowledge.

I appreciate Jack Canfield and his CEO Patty Aubery. They gave me the feedback I needed to really believe in what I was trying to accomplish with this book.

1106 Design has been instrumental in shepherding me through the publishing process. From designing the cover to picking the font to putting together the finished book. They have contributed a professionalism to this project.

I want to thank Z.La of Autonomous Art. She is an artist that drew the illustrations for this book. I had worked with several other artists but it wasn't till Z.La came along that I was able to use her creativity to find what I was looking for. And she nailed it. Thank you for working with me and being patient with me.

I have a deep gratitude for the thousands of patients and friends who had to listen to me talk about this book and its contents. They were my sounding board, my focus group, my cheerleaders and my proving grounds. I must tell you that I was attending a Tony Robbins conference and I was sobbing at the thought of having to tell my patients that I just never got this book done and published and that I had been leading them all these years. Fortunately, I can now thank them with a published book.

Anny Williams is a patient that was responsible for my author page. She was a true friend and willing to give me tough constructive criticisms that made that page much better than my original attempt.

I couldn't have finished this project if it were not for my family. My mother and stepfather, my brothers and sisters, my adult children, my adult stepchildren, and my extended family. They have provided me the supportive platform that I could count on when I was launching into territories unknown, such as going to college or medical school or residency or becoming an author. It would be my hope that everyone has the support of their family that I have enjoyed my whole life.

I want to thank Rachel Cornelio. She was my first assistant. She helped me get the ball rolling before she had to move on to another calling.

Madison is my current assistant. Her work and dedication have been a blessing. She and her family, have all contributed to this endeavor. Their input has been invaluable to getting this project completed and laying the groundwork for an organization that I envision helping people reduce their stress for the next generation and on. I've known Madison since she was 2 years old and to watch her grow from a child to a confidant, competent, hardworking young woman has been remarkable and I'm thankful she is by my side in this work.

And lastly, I want to recognize my wife Terri for the stalwart she has been. She, more than anyone else, has had to listen and read about this book. She has sacrificed her time, her attention, her expertise and, our finances to get this book to the finish line. She has been understanding of my drive to help patients even when that interrupted or completely eliminated our time together. I hope she knows how much my heart overflows with gratitude and appreciation for all she has sacrificed for this project.

Table of Contents

Introduction: Help

How Can You Help Me?
What Makes You the Expert?

*C*indy *was sitting at her cluttered desk,* anxiously asking me to sign someone's advance-directive form. I always feel like she is waiting for me to yell at her for asking for such a huge favor when, in fact, it is my *job* to sign these documents in a timely fashion. I reached across her desk to get the unsigned document, and she looked embarrassed that her desk was so messy. She explained to me she was going to clean up and organize her desk. I took a moment to assess the situation. Across from me was a 50-ish-year-old woman with whom I have worked for two years. She had always been nervous, self-deprecating, and a bit disorganized, but something had changed. She was more worried and anxious than usual. I thought she could use some help.

"Cindy, is something new bothering you?" I asked. She shuffled her papers, and a tear formed in her eye. She sighed and told me her boss had embarrassed her at a recent meeting. But she felt the boss was right about her poor performance. She went on to tell me she was always worried about losing her job,

1

her son getting into trouble with the law, and her inability to find a new significant other since she'd gotten divorced. She felt guilty about letting her boss and her son down. She regretted many of her decisions. She was just overwhelmed.

It made *me* want to cry. It was then I realized that I had the skills and knowledge to help Cindy, if she was willing. I could guide her past some of these debilitating stresses so she could be happier and more successful.

In the next 30 minutes, she told me a story of her childhood, in which her father was hurting her mother, and, at eleven years old, she felt guilty she hadn't done enough to help her mother. She told me of having a hard time paying attention and being organized. She told me her self-esteem had always been low, at best. She cried. I listened patiently and tried to put myself in her position.

When she had finished her story, I tried put her story into a new framework. I helped her reduce her guilt about her eleven-year-old self. She was surprised to feel a huge burden lifted from her chest. We worked on ways to worry less. She was willing to take a test that showed she had mild ADD, and we found an over-the-counter medicine that really helped her; she proudly told me her boss had given her a compliment at the last meeting. She was feeling less overwhelmed, more organized, more sure of herself. She was now coming to work with a smile, and she had a date with a nice man coming up soon.

It is stories like this that made me want to take this message to others like her. I realized Cindy wasn't the only one with overwhelming stress. I came to the conclusion that writing this book was the most effective way to reach as many people as I could. I want to help you find the Highway to Your Happy Place and then spend as much time in your Happy Place as you can. This book will provide you the roadmap to help you get to your destination faster and more directly.

First things first. Thank you for inviting me into your life. It has been my honor to help thousands of people in my years as a physician, and I look forward to helping you manage your stresses.

You can't see me, but I'm excited. I have been honing the concepts in this book for years and I'm now ready to share them with you. Too many people I meet are stressed out. They feel out of control. Unfortunately, they resign themselves to a life of stress. They feel like there is nothing they can do to change the current situation. They wake up every day with fear of what disaster the world will bring them today. But I am here to tell you it doesn't have to be like that.

You are amazing. You have incredible skills. You have skills that no other organism on the planet possesses. I want you to wake up in your Happy Place and go to bed in your Happy Place. I want you to regain control of your life. I want you to stop resigning yourself to living in fear and misery. Give up your learned helplessness. You have power. I learned from one of my teachers that we have the skills necessary to get what we want. It is always there within us. We just need to realize what skills we have and how to use them effectively and then take action.

This point was brought home when I read "Man's Search for Meaning" by Victor Frankl. He was a psychiatrist who was trapped in the holocaust. He was a prisoner. He was subjected to inhumane conditions with the threat of death every minute of every day. Yet he figured out that even though his situation was not under his control, his reaction to his situation was under his control. He realized that humans have the skill of hope and the power to adjust their perceptions. He made it through this miserable situation with those skills. When he wrote his book, he went to great lengths to tell his readers he did not possess any superhuman skills. He was an ordinary man using his ordinary skills. And I agree with him. We all have the power and skills within ourselves to get through the worst nightmare situation.

> One of the main themes of this book is that:
> We cannot control what happens to us, but we can control how we react to it.

You do not have to be a person with superhero skills. You can just be a regular human with regular human skills. Because regular human skills are amazing. But here is what you do need. Knowledge.

You need to know what these skills are and you need to know where all this stress originates. Only through knowledge can you hope to gain control of your stresses. When you learn where your stresses are coming from, then you can be more effective at alleviating the burden of stress and spend more time in your Happy Place.

In my original manuscripts, I placed an emphasis on having less stress. But after reading Dr Wayne Scott Andersen's book, "Dr A's Habits of Health", I realized I was ignoring the other end of the equation. If the equation is Less Stress = Happy Place. I want to emphasize the Happy Place. In Dr A's book he doesn't want you to diet to lose weight. His insight is that when you are motivated to make changes in your weight and you diet and you are successful and you lose to your goal weight, your motivation to maintain your diet is lost because you have reached your goal. When you lose your motivation, you don't continue to make the choices it took to lose the weight and consequently you gain back the weight you lost. He wants his readers to change their goal from losing weight to being healthy. When being healthy is your goal, then your motivation remains even after you have lost your weight. You still want to be healthy so you continue to make better choices.

This translates to what I am trying to accomplish. I want you to have less stress but the real reason to have less stress is so you can spend all your time in your Happy Place. I would tell patients and friends I am writing a book on how to have less stress and they would always ask for a copy so they could have less stress too. I started asking them if they had less stress where would that put them. They would get a blank look on their face. They never thought that far. Just having less stress would be so nice. But I realized people need to know where they would end up if they had less stress because this is the real goal, hence the title to this book is Highway to Your Happy Place, not Highway to Less Stress. In this book, I will show you the ingredients to what makes a Happy Place. There are at least 5 ingredients I will discuss. In each of our Happy Places there is contentment, happiness, anticipation of good things, gratitude, and fulfillment. When you have these, you will be able to enjoy life in your Happy Place.

Another main theme of this book is:
Spend as much time as you can in your Happy Place.

As I stated earlier, knowledge is important. There are so many obstacles and roadblocks to spending time in your Happy Place.

But if you don't know what the roadblocks are, how can you possibly navigate around them? And this leads to the third theme to this book. I have a secret to share with you. I have uncovered a groundbreaking new way to define where the majority of human stresses originate. This new insight will change your life.

I have reviewed hundreds of books on stress and stress reduction, and none of them look at stress the way I do. Up until now, experts defined the events and problems that cause stress. They ranked the top one hundred stresses such as death of a spouse, divorce, losing a job, etc. they give you advice on how to handle that stress. But these are external to you, and you have little control over the events and problems that you are forced to deal with during your lifetime. Sometimes they will focus on your reactions to stress and advise you to not feel angry or to love yourself no matter what. These are good recommendations but the problem is they are superficial. When I asked patients to define worry or what is an emotion, it was clear they only had a superficial response and that includes many therapists. If your definition is superficial, how effective can you be? As a doctor, when I have a better understanding of the medical problem, my solutions are much more effective. I was able to uncover the true source of stress in humans.

You're telling me that, despite thousands of books on stress, you have something NEW?

Yes, that is correct. Here it is—right in the Introduction.

Humans are amazing. We have incredible skills. We can envision the future; we can solve problems in our head; we have words and tools; we can choose between options; we can classify right and wrong, and much more. You should take a moment to appreciate the wonder of human skills.

But, there is a problem that comes with our skills. They come with side effects. For every skill that humans have, there is a side effect or downside. What I uncovered is that the majority of our stresses are a result of the side effects to our skills.

> The third main theme of this book is:
> The majority of human stress comes from the side effects to our skills.

Here is an example to clarify. You can envision the future. You see that, at some age, you want to retire. You start saving years in advance for that moment when you retire. What an amazing advantage it is to be able to envision the future. The side effect is that you have to worry about it. You can think of a hundred (or probably more) things that will get in the way of having enough money to retire. You can have a panic attack right now thinking of all the trials and tribulations you will need to go through to save enough to retire. If you couldn't envision the future, if you didn't have that amazing skill, you would have less stress, because you wouldn't be able to worry. Experts do this when they tell you not to worry or just "live for today." That implies that you must give up one of your greatest skills. Why would I want to give up a skill that has enabled the most successful species ever to exist?

> The fourth main theme of this book is:
> Keep your amazing skills and lose the side effects.

The objective of this book is for you to spend as much time as you can in your Happpy Place. To do that, you need to understand where your stresses are coming from and you need to believe you can make effective changes that will reduce your stress.

Each chapter will present a human skill and then show you the side effect. There will be six skills/stresses in this book. The six stresses are worry, guilt, regret, boredom, low self-esteem, and being overwhelmed. In each chapter, I will show you the skills that you possess as well as the side effects that occur. With this new perspective, you will have a better, more concrete understanding of where your stresses are coming from. Armed with this information, you can use the tools at the end of each chapter to reduce your stress.

That sounds good, but I need to hear more: What makes you an expert?
I have been helping the patients in my practice for 37 years. That's thousands of patient visits. During each visit, I have dealt with some aspect of a patient's stress. That's a lot of stress. I have read hundreds of books and articles, talked to many practitioners, attended conferences, and listened closely to my patients in my effort to find improved ways to identify stress and handle it more effectively. I want you to know that I am not coming at this as an outside observer. I have had my own 55-gallon drum of stress. I worked my way through college delivering newspapers at four in the morning and going to three hours of wrestling practice at four in the afternoon. Medical school was an 80-hour-a-week job. Internship was a 120-hour-a-week job. Then I had to find a job in an underserved area of the country that my wife could tolerate. We had kids. We had bills. Sometimes the income was less than the bills. My wife and I went through a bitter divorce. I have had professional problems such as a malpractice suit, troubles with the medical board, and more. Trust me, I have had my own stresses. But

the concepts and tools in this book have allowed me to spend a lot less time being stressed and more time in my Happy Place. And this book will help *you* get there, too.

I'm going to be honest with you. There are nights when I find myself in the cold sweat of fear. Who the hell am I to boldly claim I can ease your stress? My self-questioning about exactly that is probably one of the reasons this book has taken so long to come to fruition. Each time I see a patient, there is a part of me that hopes I have the skill to help. As each visit progresses, I gain confidence that all the work I have put into my profession has paid off. I *do* have something to offer the suffering patient across from me. I am neither a wizard with a magic wand nor a charlatan. What I am is a conscientious medical doctor with a strong work ethic, insight, and a genuine desire to help you.

For many patients, I have found that knowing someone listens, understands, and really wants to help them get better is half (or maybe even more) of the journey to a life of less stress. It is also important for a person to know that they are not the only one facing stress-related problems. This is important enough to repeat. *You are not alone.* When I read authors like Brené Brown and Jennie Lawson, their message is clear; lots of other people feel just the way you do. Do not isolate yourself. It's OK to ask for help. And that's why I'm here. I have worked hard to be as empathetic as possible. Through my own struggles and my research, I have come to a new and different understanding that I hope to bring to you in a way you can feel emotionally and intellectually understood.

My philosophy, as a doctor, has always been to listen attentively to my patients. My goal is that, after each visit, each patient will feel better in some way. Sometimes I can give them a clear diagnosis that gives them hope, direct them to the proper consultant, or help them navigate the red tape of the medical system. Maybe I am able to teach them about their illness or get a needed medication preauthorized. A key blood test might kickstart the trip to well-being. There is even healing in holding someone's hand, giving an empathetic hug, or sharing a joke or personal story that brings a smile to a patient with cancer. Or maybe it's all about setting the wheels in motion for counseling and guidance for a person or family member in the throes of addiction.

Or it could even be writing a book about stress. I am willing to offer anything I can to help you, my patient, feel better.

I have found that patients learn to trust their doctor over time. I hope, as we spend this time together, you will learn to trust that I have your best interests at heart. As patients learn to trust their doctor, they see the doctor as a resource for more than just their medical needs, and they are willing to share some of their most intimate fears, concerns, and needs. I realized I had a choice. I could refer my stressed-out patients to a local psychologist, knowing that many would not go because of money or some lingering bias toward the psychology field, or I could try to help my patients and use the trust they had built over time with me. It meant studying and learning and listening and exploring and risking, but this is the path I chose. It is with a passion that I have learned that, by becoming a physician to the body, brain, and mind of my patients, I have been able to become a truly holistic physician.

Calling myself *a holistic doctor* sounds weird. It's kind of like the time I shaved my head for Halloween. I wanted to look like Pitbull. The costume was a big success. The next day, I went to work at a local nursing home. I overhead a nurse tell a patient that the bald doctor would see her today. I looked around to see who she was referring to and realized she was talking about me. Oops. I wasn't used to being described as *the bald doctor*. Now my granddaughter calls me bald Pops (she is so cute). Similarly, I feel weird calling myself holistic. But I realized that is exactly what I am. One of my strengths is the fact that I am not a psychologist. I am able to balance diagnosing medical and physical problems, prescribing medications, and ordering tests with the empathy necessary for helping patients navigate the psychological struggles that come with life. I had seven brutal years of medical training but have since read as many psychological books as medical books. I have learned hypnosis and Neurolinguistic Programming. I have learned about Podiatry, Chiropractic, Raki, Psilocybin, Acupuncture, and many more therapeutic modalities—all in an effort to help you get past these energy-draining roadblocks to your Happy Place. My job is to help you navigate that Happiness Highway in any way I can.

I do realize how intimidating the medical world can be. It took me four years of medical school and three years of residency to learn the language of Medicalese. It is a foreign language to all but medically trained people. When I first started my practice in 1985, I remember seeing the glaze of incomprehension come across a patient's face when I explained how the islet cells of the pancreas make insulin to lower your body's glucose level. Fortunately, it didn't take me long to realize my patients had no clue as to what I was talking about.

That realization added to my job as a physician. I had to make the complicated medical world as understandable as I could. To do that, I draw pictures, make analogies, open illustrated books, point to models, Google images, use more common terms, and watch for signs of information overload. In this book, I will use all the tools I can to help you understand the concepts you need to know and how you can incorporate them into your life. As I have learned from my many teachers, if you don't understand what I am saying, then I didn't say it correctly for you.

I also am not afraid to share my life, my experiences, and my mistakes with my patients. In this way, I make our visit a two-way encounter. My patients are more willing to share with me when I am willing to share with them. I have had my share of stresses, and, like all people, I am a work in progress. Believe me when I say this: If not for my circle of family, friends, and patients, I would be in a much worse state. And there's one other thing that helped me: I read my book. Why write a book for others if you don't use the principles and strategies yourself?

It is against this backdrop that I chose to write this book. I have a desire to help the patients who come to my office, the patients I treat face to face. But I also have a desire to help the millions of other people who are suffering from too much stress and unable to find their Happy Place. This book culminates more than three decades as a doctor and twenty-five years of focused study on stress-related problems and their solutions.

By the end of this book, you should be able to appreciate what marvelous creatures humans are. You will be able to identify and understand where our human skills come from and then identify the side effects to these skills. You will have lots of tools to use to reduce or eliminate the side effects and still be able to keep the skills. You will be able to grasp where your Happy Place is and what the ingredients are to a Happy Place. This book cannot take away all your stresses, but it can give you a way to manage them more effectively and efficiently.

That is why I think I am qualified to help you with your stress. I really hope you believe me and read on. I really want to help you get to your Happy Place and stay there as long as you can.

There are four "housekeeping" points I want to make.

Point 1: Definitions matter. How you define a concept makes a huge difference in how you communicate about that concept. Those things, in turn, influence how effective a solution will be. I have spent a lot of time trying to precisely define the words and concepts I use in the book so that you will be clear on what I am trying to say. For example, when I talk to worried patients in my practice, I ask them to define "worry." They get a confident smile and begin their definition, but it doesn't take long before they realize that it's easy to use "worry" in a sentence or identify "worry" when they see it (or, more likely, feel it), but that defining "worry" is not so easy.

The same is true for professionals. Here is an example to illustrate my point. In the past, doctors didn't really know how to define diabetes beyond *a patient had too much sugar in their system.* Doctors would dab patients' urine on their tongues; if it tasted sweet, the diagnosis was diabetes. (Fortunately for me, we have better diagnostic tools now.) As medical knowledge expanded, we learned to define diabetes as a condition in which there was not enough insulin, or a resistance to insulin, or unregulated glucagon or gastric hormones, or defective insulin-transport mechanisms. As our definition became more precise, so did our tests and treatments. I have practiced long enough to see the revolution that has occurred in how we care for patients with diabetes.

In this book, I will provide you the best definition I can for each problem. I want to be able to use the definition's detail to help dig deep into the problem and uncover the most effective ways to treat it. The definitions I use may not be the definitions you use. However, once you hear and understand my definitions, I hope the treatments I offer at the end of each chapter will make sense. Identifying and understanding a problem makes solving it a lot easier.

Point 2: I want to make an underlying theme very clear before there are misinterpretations that make people angry. Humans are, first, biological organisms. There are functions that any organism must perform successfully to stay alive: Find food, shelter, and water; reproduce; interact with the environment; stay safe; and so forth. We share these functions with every other organism, even if we problem-solve in different ways.

Humans are primates, and there are many patterns that we share with other primates. However, there are also patterns we do not share, largely because most primates evolved as berry-and-nut eaters, while humans evolved as hunters. Even though our primate patterns overlapped with the behaviors of a hunter, our brains haven't lost their primate urges (at least, not yet). These patterns and behaviors can clash.

If that's not enough, we added another wrinkle: directed awareness (which I define later in the book). Directed awareness led to communication, technology, the creation of societies, and other advancements. It also led to conflict. That happens when our societal rules run afoul of our biological goals. China's one-child policy is a good example. When China launched a population-control policy that restricted every family to having just one child, it created an enormous conflict with the biological drive behind our reproductive behavior.

Throughout this book, I try to differentiate between what is biological and what is societal, but that distinction some-times gets prickly. If something in this book starts to raise your hackles, remember that I come from a biological point of view. (A good book that discusses this is Desmond Morris's *The Naked Ape*.)

Point 3: As you read my book, I want you to think of yourself as a student. A student must be willing to listen, to learn, and to incorporate new ideas into their life. A student must be able to admit they don't know everything. A student must be willing to climb out of the rut that has been burrowed over the years and step onto a new path. This is scary and disruptive, but it is essential if you really want to change. Jack Canfield tells his readers they will experience fear, but that, to be successful, you need to take action *anyway*. Another way to say that is *Bravery is not the **absence** of fear, but taking action **despite** your fear.* Less stress won't happen without change. Make the commitment to read the rest of this book with an open-to-change mindset.

The corollary to you being a student is that I have to be a good teacher or coach. That means I must find a way for you to understand the information I am sharing. It also means that I treat you with the respect and empathy you deserve. Together, as student and teacher, we can accomplish a lot.

Point 4: This book is written for a general audience. It cannot be individualized. That is not what I am used to. As a physician, I usually work the other way around. I take general information and personalize it to you. So, if you have a specific question about your situation, you can reach me through my website, *The Less Stress Doc.com.*

Every question is important. My goal is for you to have less stress and more time in your Happy Place. If there is something you don't understand, let me know, so that I can help you.

Now get into the car, and let's drive on the Happiness Highway and get to your destination Happy Place. The first step is finding your place on the map.

CHAPTER ONE

Stress/Less Stress

How Bad Is It? How Good Could It Be?

In this chapter, I will describe "being stressed." I will detail the amazing skills we have as humans. I will explain that the majority of human stress is a side effect of our human skills. I will begin the process of showing you how to reduce the side effect and keep the skill. I will introduce you to a new tool called Stratasphers. I will show you how understanding the mind/brain connection will make it easier for you to see where your stresses are coming from. I will define what a Happy Place looks like. There are five components to everyone's Happy Place.

You are at the entrance ramp to your Happiness Highway. Here you are at the red X. YOU ARE HERE. This is the place where you have more stress than you can manage, and finding your Happy Place is proving nearly impossible. No doubt you're wondering, "How the hell did I get here?"

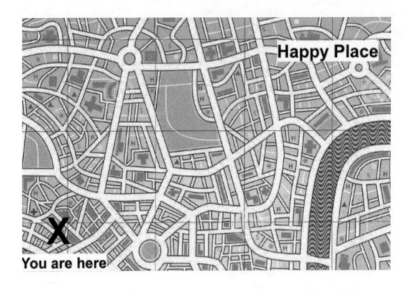

I have seen thousands of patients just like you, so I know that YOU ARE HERE is a scary place. You are frightened, worried, and overwhelmed. Problems are coming at you faster than you can fix them. You feel that the battle is constant, you're not winning, and no end appears in sight. There are no solutions that make sense for you, and it is hard to ask for help when you have so much on your plate already. You have resigned yourself to always being stressed out. Please don't give up. There is a way to be less stressed. You have already taken a step by getting this book.

Don't resign yourself to to a stressed-out life. There is an achievable alternative.

I want to repeat this point. You don't have to live a stressed-out life. It is not inevitable, and it is not unalterable. The reason I can guarantee that you will feel less stress is because once you understand where your stresses are coming from and some concrete actions you can take, you will feel less stressed. Your stresses will become more manageable; you will spend less time overwhelmed and in fear and spend more time in your Happy Place—a place where you will feel contentment and fulfillment. It is not an imaginary place. It is for real, and you can be there for the majority of your life. All it takes is some understanding coupled with some action.

You might have tried other avenues before you called me. I'm going to guess they didn't help—or I wouldn't be here with you. You can't afford to waste your energy on things that don't work because you barely have enough energy to keep yourself above the tidal wave of stressors. Your physiology is being pushed into overdrive. Your danger response is kicking in constantly. You can't sleep. Stomach ulcers are forming.

You get the point. More than that, you *live* the point. (A helpful book about our body's response to stress is *Why Zebras Don't Get Ulcers,* by Robert M. Sapolsky.) Our bodies respond to stress in countless ways. And we are seeing the consequences to those responses. Addiction, suicide, and psychiatric illness are at all-time highs. Burnout is so prevalent that it is hard to find someone who isn't. People have lost their hope that things will get better because they are inundated with all the things that go wrong. There has to be a better way to stop all this stress. I believe there is; if I didn't, this book would be a waste of your time.

Let's start with the upside. To be human is amazing. That's right—humans are *amazing*. Our supremacy on the Earth is unparalleled. Soak that in for a second. Pat yourself on the back if you are human. An average human's skill set is incomprehensible to every other animal that exists on this planet. Here are some particular skills we have as humans.

The human ability to learn is breathtaking.

There is an experiment I always wished my kids would have done for their 6th-grade science fair. It involves timing how long it takes to teach a guinea pig to sit on command, how long it takes a dog to learn that command, and how long it takes a two-year-old child. Unfortunately, my kids never took up my suggestion, so I can't say for sure, but my guess is that it would take a guinea pig days—if ever. It might take a dog hours. But a human child would get the skill in seconds. Incredible. In seconds, a young, unsophisticated child can learn a complex activity that most animals would never master, and those that could accomplish the task would require days of laborious training.

Another marvelous thing that humans can do is envision the future.

We can make a reasonable guess about the near future and make or change our plans to ensure a good outcome. What other animal has anywhere near this capability? Maybe an orca whale or an elephant has some sense of the future, but a human's capability in this area dramatically dwarfs that. We can look into next week, next year, even the next century, and beyond. In fact, looking forward to the future has become so much a part of our lives that humans *can't live for today* even if they tried.

Choice—the ability to select or make a decision when there are multiple possibilities—is another amazing skill that is quintessentially human.

We can eat chocolate ice cream or broccoli. We can plan a night at the movies or decide to go the football game. We can ask someone to the prom or go stag. Some animals are capable of rudimentary choice, but most animals must do what their brain tells them. If a lion is hungry, she will hunt an antelope. If she is not hungry, she will sit in the sun. She does not choose what or where to eat, how to prepare it, or how to store it. A human's ability to choose is so far beyond that of other animals that it is fair to say we are the only organism that has real decision-making power.

Humans have another power that eludes animals. Humans can distinguish right from wrong.

Other organisms can be taught not to do something, but humans take this concept to a whole new level. Humans have unwritten rules, as well as tomes of written rules and laws, that lay out which actions and intentions are right and which are wrong. This skill allows us to have peaceful societies. It allows people the ability (even if not currently realized) to live together without strife on a planet that now supports billions of human lives.

Unlike the vast majority of animals, humans have self-image.

Newborns can't distinguish "us" from "them." But as babies grow and develop, it doesn't take long before they can. Like the rest of us, children can recognize themselves in a mirror. Older humans use that mirror to make themselves more attractive. We can dress up for Halloween and alter our self-image as needed. A chameleon can only change color. We can change our height, our voice, our clothes, our skin. Watch any sci-fi movie to see how scriptwriters and actors play with that concept.

Humans have the unique ability to use tools.

I'm writing this book with the aid of a computer, sitting in my house that was built with hammers and electric saws, using materials that were brought by trucks. The number of tools we can use is almost limitless. And we can learn to use them in minutes (sometimes).

Language is another astonishing human attribute.

Of course, other organisms can communicate—honks, whistles, oinks, neighs, screeches, clicks. But how much detail can be conveyed in this form of communication? Humans can express words and concepts. We can communicate about things that are in the room as well as things that don't even exist. We can write a book that a million people can read. And twenty years from now, a million people in a new generation can read the same book and receive the same message.

Our curiosity is unprecedented among fauna, or, heck, even flora.

We are driven to explore new areas, new ideas, new tools, new relationships. Solitary confinement is one of the worst punishments we have devised because it strangles the ability to exercise one's curiosity. Is it any surprise that solitary confinement can cause mental illness? My dog will sniff a crab. One pinch, and his curiosity is satisfied—and he keeps his distance. But a human who sees a crab may want to know everything they can about it—where it lives, what it eats, how to catch it and not get pinched, how it mates, what its genes look like, and on and on. We are insatiable when it comes to curiosity.

I repeat for emphasis: Humans are *amazing*.

We are the dominant species on earth. Lions, ha. Tigers, pshaw. A COVID virus tried to take us down and, in less than a year, we figured out how to neutralize it. We can feed 7 billion people. We can identify and cure many illnesses. We can tame other animals and have them do things for us. We can build dams or even carve statues out of mountainsides. We can live underwater and fly into space. Our skills make us the most adaptable organism on the planet.

But (and it's a really big but) there is a downside. And that's where the trouble begins.

Each skill we have comes with, as we say in my doctor world, a side effect. Each skill we have gives us a great benefit, but it also can cause problems. If I give a patient a medication for high blood pressure, it carries the benefit that it brings down their blood pressure. It also carries a potential side effect of making the patient tired or swollen or depleted of potassium. If a patient comes to my office with pneumonia, I can pick from a menu of treatments. Each treatment has a benefit and a side effect. If I pick an antibiotic that you are allergic to, it will fix your respiratory infection, but you will break out in a rash from head to toe. Not all the side effects are physical. If I pick an antibiotic that is too expensive for your budget, you might have the side effect of not having enough money to pay your rent this month.

In my practice, I work very hard to find treatments that carry a maximum benefit with the minimum number of side effects. Indeed, it has been helpful for me to look at the whole world through this lens of benefits and side effects. There is value in training yourself to think this way, to think like a doctor. When you are trying to decide whether to commute to work by train or take your own car, you can think of the benefits and side effects of each choice. This helps lead to an informed decision.

When I started looking at human stresses, it dawned on me that the majority of human stress is really the downside or side effect of some of our amazing human skills.

I reread the books on stress and found that most authors detail a person's response to stress. Or they list or rank external stresses in some sort of order. Or they provide people with a generic prescription to meditate or exercise. But no one has looked at our stresses as the side effect or downside to our skills. This realization is what drove me to write this book. This is the insight that gives us a better understanding of how we got to YOU ARE HERE. This is the insight that points us to the specific tools we need to counteract the side effects of stress. This is the insight that will help you find your Happy Place and eliminate the obstacles en route.

> The majority of human stress is a side effect or downside to our amazing skills.

Let that sink in for a minute.
It's worth repeating.

> The majority of human stress is a side effect or downside to our amazing skills.

Can you give me an example of what you are talking about?

Sure. We have a number of skills that have enabled us to be the dominant species on Earth. These skills have made us a biological success story. But each skill can also cause problems. Let's think about our skill of envisioning the future. We can see a hurricane coming and prepare ahead of time for the dangerous weather that is about to strike. We can run to higher ground, board up the house, put sandbags around our foundation. If we have enough warning, we can drive miles away from the storm or build levees. This is the upside. We can envision the future and make changes in our lives that bring about a more desirable outcome.

The downside is that, to be ready to act, we also have to worry about the future. We envision being trapped in a flooded house without electricity, running water, or food. We imagine a loved one drowning in hurricane floodwaters. We picture our house destroyed and all our heirlooms and family treasures washed away. These disastrous images in our head fire up our emotions. We shake in fear, we cry, we get angry, we get sad. We feel horrible, we feel stressed out. There is nothing to stop these terrible thoughts. They just keep popping into our heads, over and over again, triggering draining emotional responses.

My patients with dementia and my newborn granddaughter cannot envision the future. They don't have that skill. When you can't envision the future, you can't worry about the future, and, consequently, you have a lot less stress. But without the skill of envisioning the future, you probably won't survive the hurricane.

This pattern is repeated with our other skills. Each skill we have as a human has a potential side effect. When you look at our stresses from this point of view, then the real questions are, "What skills do humans have?" "What are the side effects of these skills?" and "How do we get rid of the side effects and keep the skills?"

How can I keep my amazing skills and get rid of—or at least diminish—the side effects or downside?

This is the whole crux of this book: Understanding that the reason humans are so stressed is the same reason we are so successful. Our skills are amazing, but side effects pull us away from our Happy Place.

> Figuring out a way to eliminate or reduce the side effects and still keep our skills is why I wrote this book.

The wording of this statement is key. It values the upside of being human, acknowledges the downside, and looks for a possible route to our Happy Place. We need our skills. Many mental-health professionals will advise you to just *live for today*, but that implies giving up one of the best skills we have as humans: the ability to envision the future. It is the skill that allows us to survive the hurricane. I don't want to stop planning for the future. I want to keep my skill but lose the side effect.

The premise of this book (and others to follow) is that humans have amazing skills that have side effects, and the recommendations I suggest for you are based on the idea of keeping our skills and losing the side effects. Once you start thinking of your stresses as side effects to your skills, then finding ways to have less stress gets easier and more efficient. This insight makes it easier to dodge the obstacles that are blocking your entrance to the Happiness Highway and finding your Happy Place.

How did you come up with this perspective?

I didn't start out pondering the question *How can I alleviate all the stresses of human life?* In fact, I didn't start out to answer *any* question. I was reading an eclectic array of books, from physics to anthropology; from self-help to mathematics; sociology, psychology, medical; marketing and advertising, from philosophy to religion. I learned a little something from each book, but it wasn't until I discovered Strataspheres that it all started making sense. "Discovered" is probably not the right word. What I really did was pull together good, but isolated, ideas from the books I read to create a new tool. This tool provided me a framework or template into which I could insert information and then gain a new insight.

My template/tool is called Strataspheres. I could go into great detail about this template (and, believe me, the readers of my book's first drafts will tell you I did), but, with the wisdom of retrospection, I will keep it brief. Think of Strataspheres as layered spheres. There is a core; then new layers are wrapped around the core. Here is a picture of what I am describing.

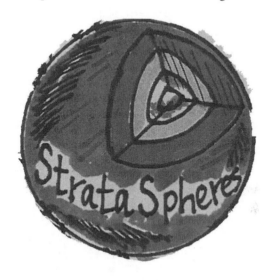

(In Appendix One, there is a more complete description of Strataspheres.)

What makes Strataspheres so important is that it helps us understand how humans got to be so different than other organisms. It shows how we got to be so dominant. But it also shows how we got to be so stressed out. One insight of Strataspheres is explaining how we got a mind from a bunch of neurons. Lots of other animals have a brain with neurons and axons, but humans have an emergent skill set that is the mind. It is the mind skills that have set us apart, and Strataspheres helps us understand how the mind came to exist. It also shows why some humans have a brain but don't have a mind.

Take a newborn. An infant has a brain, and that brain has all the same characteristics as my brain. Infants know how to cry, how to eat, how to grab a finger or a mother's boob. But newborns can't envision the future. Newborns can't talk. Newborns don't have self-awareness. Newborns can't think. Newborns don't have a concept of right and wrong or good and bad. The reason for this is that they don't have enough neurons or connections. They haven't crossed the threshold. They have a brain but don't have a mind—yet.

As a human baby develops, more neurons are made, more connections are formed, and the emergent properties of a mind appear.

Now let's go to the other end of the spectrum. I am a prima-ry-care doctor who visits patients in nursing homes. Many of those patients have dementia. (In this example, I am referring to end-stage patients, not early-onset patients.) These patients have a brain. If you do computerized tomography (CT) scans, their brains will appear a little shriveled, but there is no CT scan that differentiates a patient with dementia from a patient who doesn't have dementia. Nonetheless, the skill set is very different. Patients with dementia can cry, can eat, can grab things (and yes, nurses will tell you they can grab a boob). Patients with dementia can walk and vocalize. But they don't have a concept of the future. They can't think. They can't rea-son. They don't have self-awareness. They have lost the outer sphere of mind.

There is no one event that leads to this loss. It is a slow, inter-mittent, back-and-forth process. There are some good days and some bad days but the slope is downward, as the patient loses skills and doesn't get them back. When the dementia patient loses enough brain cells and/or connections, a threshold is re-crossed, and the emergent properties of mind disappear. The dementia patient no longer has a mind or the skills that go with it.

Our mind is what separates us from other animals, so it is no wonder that most humans fear dementia more than they fear death.

How does this connect to stress?

Because newborns and dementia patients don't have a mind, they also have a lot less stress than you or I do. They don't envision the future and worry if there will be food to eat tomorrow or who will pay the bills if the breadwinner loses their job. They don't feel guilty if screaming for hours keeps others awake. They don't get embarrassed that the clothes they have on clash or are unfashionable. They don't look in the mirror and grow concerned about their skin or lack of hair or lack of teeth. Their life is much simpler. They do what medical professionals have told us how to be less stressed. They *live for today.*

They have a lot less stress, but, unfortunately, they are also a lot less successful. They can't live independently in our world. They would die. They don't have enough skills to get food or water or shelter. They need a human who has a mind to care and provide for them.

This is why Strataspheres matters. When you realize how you got a mind and that your mind is what differentiates you from other animals, you then can recognize that the majority of your stress is because of those mind skills. The biggest sources of stress, as you will learn throughout this book, are *side effects* of those mind skills. With that understanding, you have a better roadmap, and you can identify the obstacles blocking the entrance to your Happiness Highway and your Happy Place destination.

You can start to see how, despite having the best standard of living ever in the history of mankind, we are the most stressed civilization that has ever existed. It is largely because the emergent properties of the mind have side effects that humans are led into being the most stressed organism in existence. YOU ARE HERE is because you have a brain and a mind. Your mind is a set of skills, and the skills have side effects. The side effects lead you to being stressed out. The only way to have less stress is to understand what skills you have and find ways to reduce the side effects.

That's interesting, but what I really want to hear about is the destination. Tell me about my Happy Place: How do I get there and spend the rest of my life there?

I learned from my book consultant, Steve Harrison, and his wife, Laura Harrison, that readers don't want to spend time learning the mechanics of the boat that takes them across the river. They just want to get to the other side, where the fun is. What is a Happy Place? If we can't answer that question, then how can we get there and enjoy the wonderful life we envision?

"Happy Place" is really a vague term. But its vagueness is actually helpful. It can be individualized. *You* get to identify what your Happy Place is. Your Happy Place is probably very different from my Happy Place. But since we are using the same map to get there, I need to find common landmarks or highway signs that will enable you to realize you have reached your destination—your Happy Place.

Here's what I have found about a Happy Place: Even though it can be different for each individual, there are some common characteristics. I have identified at least five distinct and separate ingredients that define a Happy Place: Contentment, Happiness, Anticipation of Pleasure, Gratitude and Fulfillment.

Can you give me more detail about these components?

The first component of your Happy Place—Contentment—is the balance of good and bad emotions that leads to a baseline feeling of contentment or peace.

Every person has a level of contentment that they feel at a given moment. This level fluctuates, but this is where you spend most of your emotional time. It is a balance between you feeling good and you feeling bad, depending on the circumstances you find yourself in—or, probably more important, your *perception* of the circumstances you find yourself in. Feeling bad might predominate, or feeling good might predominate. These two polar opposites pull your baseline contentment up or down. I am guessing that most people who are reading this book have a low level of contentment (Spoiler alert—it is raisable). If you're feeling anxious or sad, that pulls your contentment down. If you are excited and joyous, that pulls your contentment up.

I was trying to come up with an analogy. I was going to use muscle tone, but that seemed to appeal only to medical people, so I am going to talk about a paycheck. Think of your paycheck. You receive a regular weekly income from your job (hopefully). The weekly paycheck is the usual amount of money you get for doing a certain amount of work. Your paycheck can fluctuate any given week because you put in more hours or fewer, or you added a second job. The smaller your paycheck, the fewer things you can afford. Your choices are limited. There is more pressure on you to be able to pay your bills, and this makes you less happy. The opposite is also true. If your paycheck is higher, there is more fun in your life. There is less pressure when it comes time to pay bills. You have more choices in your life. You are happier. Contentment is like your weekly paycheck.

Your baseline can change. To continue the analogy, let's say that you get a raise. Your baseline rises. Ooops—you are forced to take a lower-paying job. Your baseline shifts downward. The baseline is fluid. The good news is that your baseline is changeable. There are things you can do to raise your baseline. Ask for a raise, take a second job, etc.

One thing to remember about contentment is that it is very dependent on your perceptions. Two people could have the same level of good and bad forces in their life, but if their perceptions are quite different, consequently, their level of contentment is different. We will talk more about perceptions later in the book. But the good news is that perceptions can be changed, and your level of contentment can go up without changing your environment—just by changing your perceptions.

Let's look at the second component—Happiness.

To define Happiness, I want to use Desmond Morris's definition. Happiness is a spike of pleasurable emotions you feel when there is an event that is making your life better. You see your newborn infant for the first time; your team wins the Super Bowl; you get accepted to the college of your dreams. Each carries a huge spike in emotion that floods you with exhilaration.

This definition implies that happiness is temporary. It is temporary because it hinges on the change from your baseline emotional state. Your contentment is the baseline of pleasure that you feel on a typical day in your life. Happiness is when there is a pleasurable change from your usual day. To go back to our paycheck analogy, your weekly paycheck is your baseline. A raise is a measurable increase in the level of your happiness. You don't get a raise every day. It is a temporary change. If the raise is permanent, then your level of contentment will go up, but the spike of happiness will melt back to the new level of contentment. If it is a one-time bonus, your happiness will go up for that time, but then you go back to your baseline paycheck and your baseline level of contentment.

Your baseline level of contentment does affect how great a change there is in your happiness. For example, if you are already in a good place and contented, a spike of happiness might not be as noticeable. If you are making $1 million a year and someone gives you a $1,000 raise, it won't have the same effect on you as it makes on someone who is making $10,000 a year. That person is getting a substantial increase from the baseline, and, consequently, their happiness will be much higher from the same amount of extra money.

In the movie *Castaway*, the main character is on a deserted island by himself. When he finally figures out how to make a fire, he is ecstatic. He jumps for joy. For me, if I want to cook a hamburger, all I have to do is light a match and I have a fire. My happiness is much less than that of the marooned man on the island, because my baseline happiness exists at a much higher tier. As the baseline rises and falls, it is the sudden upswing that causes happiness. That memory of the moment when you saw your newborn for the first time will still make you feel happy, but not nearly as strongly as when the event occurred. Happiness tends to melt back to your baseline.

There are multiple ways that a person can change their baseline contentment with happiness. One important point about Happiness is that there is an aspect of *tolerance*. If you get a bonus every month, the level of change is reduced over time. The first bonus will bring a big smile to your face and lead you to excitedly telling your spouse about the extra money. But if every month you get the same bonus, eventually the bonus melts back to your baseline, and you start to expect the bonus. You don't come home with excitement to tell your spouse. In fact, now, if you *don't* get a bonus, you get sad or angry.

Recapping, the first component is your baseline of contentment—the balance of good emotions and bad emotions in your life. The second component is the temporary change in baseline that comes from a pleasurable event.

Let's add the third component of your Happy Place—Anticipation of Pleasure.

Humans spend a lot of time in the future—looking forward to driving a car, to getting married, to having a child, to retiring. We make a lot of plans focused on the future. One of the characteristics of our Happy Place is the anticipation of something good ahead. For happiness or contentment to occur, something has to happen. But that is not the case with anticipation. It only needs us to *think* something good will happen.

I have a favorite restaurant, and I can anticipate the taste and smell of the food. It sends a pleasurable signal through my brain. When I go to the restaurant, the actual eating of the food will give me happiness over my baseline, but that may last only 30 minutes or an hour. The *anticipation* of eating the meal can be hours and days. In a lot of ways, anticipation can be more important to humans than actual happiness. I have spent years envisioning myself as a successful author who has helped thousands of suffering, stressed-out people. I get a big jolt of pleasure every time I think of that scenario. That has been going on for twenty-five years. The time you spend anticipating that good things will happen is giving you flashes of happiness that *are not based in reality.* But the feeling is real. People who anticipate that good things are coming will be physically happier, and they have also been proven to be healthier.

The next component is Gratitude. I added this component after attending a Tony Robbins seminar. He had a great point. When you are filled with gratitude, it is impossible to feel anger. You are happier when you appreciate everything you have, all the people you are connected to, and all that others have done for you. I get a happy tear in my eye when I spend time thinking about all the things people have done for me to get me to where am I am today. As much as I would like to describe myself as a self-made man, that is so far from the truth that it is delusional. There are my parents and siblings, my teachers and coaches, my professors and fellow students, my staff and patients, my business partners, my pets, my enemies, and my foes. They have all influenced my life in some way. I actually spend a lot of time feeling gratitude for the role others have played in my life. It fills me with awe and puts a giant grin on my face when I realize how much others have helped me. Sometimes they don't even know they have helped me or to the extent that they have helped. When you feel gratitude or appreciation, it makes you feel good. Hence, it is included in the definition of your Happy Place.

The last component is Fulfillment. This is also courtesy of Tony Robbins. You can have money, success, and friends—and still not feel fulfilled. You can be a multimillionaire and feel empty. You can be a tremendous performer or athlete and not feel fulfilled. You can be a great employee for thirty years and not feel fulfilled. Being fulfilled takes something else.

Being fulfilled comes from two places—growing and giving. Growing means you are learning and using your new knowledge to change the trajectory of your life. One of the reasons being a doctor is so fulfilling is that you are constantly learning and growing. I was taking care of patients with stress-reducer loops (my term for addiction). There was something missing in my treatment plans. I took it upon myself to learn about hypnosis and Neurolinguistic Programming. I learned something new, I grew as a physician, and I used the knowledge to help my patients. My patients were better because of my growth, and I had a feeling of fulfillment. Growth can take many forms. It can be learning a new skill or perfecting a skill you already have. It can be in the form of self-awareness or empathy for others. It can be reading a book of science fiction or historical fiction. Growth is essential to humans. Tony Robbins is quoted as saying, "If you don't grow, you die." I don't know if that is literally true, but it sures feels like it when you get stuck in a deep rut.

The second place is giving. When you focus on giving to others, you feel better about yourself. This is what makes being a parent so rewarding. You make someone else in your life a priority. I tell my patients you know you're a parent when you are sick with flu and feel horrible, and, yet, you make the effort to take care of your child. And that makes you feel good about yourself.

I have had the privilege of serving my patients since 1985. I have had many patients tell me how I improved their life, but one memory especially sticks out. My office decided we would reach out to our neediest family for Christmas. The staff and I picked up our family of four. To make it special, we picked them up in a limo. We went to the local department store, and they had a $500 shopping spree. The kids were young teenagers. I expected them to run to the toy department. Was I wrong! They went to the shoe department, where they got their first pair of new shoes. They picked out a blanket, so that they didn't have to use newspapers when grandmom stayed over, and they picked out a gift for their parents. The parents bought new clothes, so that they had something nice to wear when they went to church. After the shopping, we had a sit-down dinner at a local restaurant. I have no idea how much I spent in dollars that night, but my staff, my wife, and I have never felt so fulfilled. The family we helped thought they had been given a gift. What they didn't realize was that *we* were the ones that had been given a gift—a gift that will always be there in our memories.

Now we have the five components of our Happy Place. It is a combination of baseline contentment, the spikes of happiness from real events, the anticipation of pleasurable events in the future, gratitude for what you have, and feeling fulfilled through growth and giving. The more you have of these five components, the more time you get to spend in your Happy Place.

What I have found is there are specific blockages keeping you away from your Happy Place. That is where the rest of this book is focused. What are the issues that are keeping you from being contented, having pleasurable events, anticipating more, feeling gratitude, and feeling fulfilled? My contention is that the majority of blockages come from the side effects to your human mind skills.

As you read this book, keep in mind the Law of Attraction. Jack Canfield writes about this in his book *The Success Principles*. What you think about, talk about, believe strongly about, and feel intensely about—you will *bring about*. This is the beginning of you thinking about yourself as a less-stressed person who is living in your Happy Place. The tools in this book will help you achieve that goal.

The rest of this book will go into six stresses that are blocking your entrance to the Happiness Highway and arriving at your Happy Place. The following chapters will show you how to eliminate or reduce your stress so that you can spend more time in your Happy Place. *Yeaahhhhh!*

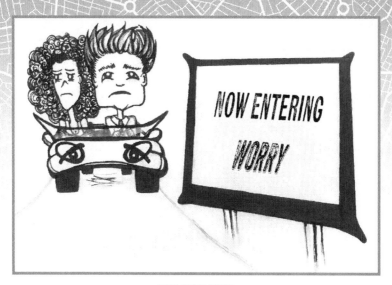

CHAPTER TWO

Worry

Is Your Danger Response Working Overtime?

In this chapter, I will define worry. I will tell you about Mary, who worries a lot. I will tell you about the skill of envisioning the future and then show you how worry is the side effect to that skill. Then I will give you some tools to alleviate worry: Realistic Optimism, Worry Organizer, Exercise, Meditation, Medication, Neurolinguistic Programming. At the end, there will be a recap.

Definition of Worry: Worry is using your mind skill of looking into the future, focusing on the bad things that could happen, and having a danger response in the present.

Mary is a patient of mine who came into the office with all the signs of significant stress. She told me she was worried all the time and that it was taking its toll on her health. Her interactions with her family were strained because worry was reducing her patience and tolerance. I asked what she was worried about. She told me she was worried she would get breast cancer. She had good reason to worry. Her mother and sister both had breast cancer.

Further, she was worried that if she was diagnosed with breast cancer, she would die and leave her husband a widower and her children without a mother. Mary looked at me with tears in her eyes and asked:

Can you help me not to worry?

Yes.

Worry is, by far, the most common stress that exists for humans. It is insidious. And it takes a physical and mental toll on the worrier. A worried patient will often tell me they are worried that they worry too much. I nod in affirmation. Yes, you are worrying too much.

The first challenge patients have is with their definition (or lack of definition) for worry. As I discussed in Chapter 1, it is really hard to fix a problem if you cannot define it or have only a superficial definition. That's why I ask worriers to define worry. I think patients are surprised by just how difficult it can be to define the word, even though they can certainly recognize the feeling that goes along with worry.

Often patients have an idea in their head of what worry is, but their definition is very nonspecific. After patients give me a definition, I ask if that definition seems useful in helping them fix their problem with worry. What they realize is that their definition connects to a concern that seems unfixable. That conundrum also explains why people—even experts—give standard advice like "Don't worry, be happy" or "Live for today" or "Don't sweat the small stuff." I suppose this advice might work for those few who can *actually* "live for today," but most humans cannot. More than half our energy is spent envisioning the future and planning for it. Envisioning the future allows us to change now to bring about desired outcomes or to avoid unwanted ones.

More importantly, "living for today" is equivalent to saying *Give up your mind skill of looking into the future.* I don't want you to give up your awesome mind skill of envisioning the future. It is one of the keys to human success, and you need it to function in any human society. What you want to give up, instead, is the *side effect* that *comes with* our amazing ability to envision the future.

| Worry is the side effect of the mind skill of envisioning the future. |

I've explained that worry comes out of our wonderful and useful ability to anticipate the future. How exactly *do* humans envision the future? This is an important question, because the answer points us toward ways to have less worry.

I just finished reading the book *The 12 Rules of Life: An Antidote to Chaos,* by Jordan Peterson. The author makes an interesting point. When you drive a car, you don't need to know how the engine works until it doesn't. Then, if you don't know how an engine works, you will be stuck on the side of the road, waiting for someone who does. I think this same idea applies to many of the topics we will discuss in this book. Currently, we are discussing the future. If you don't know how we have developed the skill to envision the future, you'll be stuck when that skill isn't working. So let me take a few paragraphs to explain how I think we envision the future.

Envisioning the future relies on our ability to recognize patterns and make models. Recognizing patterns involves examining information and finding consistent or recurring themes. If you take the pattern you find and make it into a model, you are then able to manipulate the model in various ways. Being able to find a pattern, create a model, and use that model is one of the skills that has made humans so successful.

Once I have a functional model, I can run it forward or backward, looking for answers from the past or forming predictions for the future. Let's say I have worked for a year, and, at the end of every two-week period of work, I receive a paycheck. That is a pattern. I can now look into the future and predict that I will get a paycheck at the end of a two-week period. I could look four weeks into the future or forty weeks into the future. However, the further you go into the future, the more variables that come into play—making the prediction more difficult and less accurate. Maybe I'll get sick in Week Thirty-Two. Maybe my wife will get sick, and I can't work. Maybe a hurricane will level the building where I am working. The further out you take your model, the less reliable the model's foundational information is.

As a doctor, I trained for eleven years in school and four decades of experience in private practice. I am getting better and better at recognizing the pattern that tells me a patient has diabetes or allergies or asthma or Lyme disease. I have seen these problems before. After referring to books, consultants, and the internet, I can formulate a plan on how to help alleviate the problem. That plan often involves the future.

In fact, I spend a lot of time telling patients what is going to happen in the future. If you continue to eat sugar and your blood sugar stays high, you will be more likely to have a heart attack or stroke, or lose a leg. If you have strep throat and you take this medicine, your sore throat with disappear in less than seven days. If you have cancer, you will have this long to live.

Envisioning the future is important. Being able to accurately predict what will happen allows us to change what we do today. If I want to retire, I need to save my money today so there will be enough money when I stop working. If a hurricane is coming, I need to put plywood over my windows. We are always trying to find better ways of predicting what will happen. We improve our pattern recognition, make stronger models, and run them forward in tests to see how well they work at predicting the future. We use feedback to tweak the patterns and models in order to better predict what will happen. The more accurate the predictions, the more likely we are to be successful and, in turn, the more we trust the models to give us reliable information.

Who spends 95 percent of their time in the future? Weather forecasters. The weatherman tries to tell us what the weather will be later today, tomorrow, next Saturday, next month. How does the forecaster do it? By using equipment to detect patterns, using the patterns to make models, and running those models into the future. Over the years, weather forecasting equipment has improved by leaps and bounds. Weather satellites, Doppler radar, and other advances make the data more accurate. Computer advances have made it easier to construct models, including models with more variables. The model can be run over and over, using improved information, better pattern recognition, and more refined models in order to give us more precise weather predictions.

Think how accurate the weatherman has to be. If it is 33 degrees, it will rain. If it is 31 degrees, it will snow. I can't distinguish between those two degrees, but their deviation means the difference between rain and snow. That, in turn, decides whether I can drive to work or have to shovel my driveway. I am always impressed that the weather forecaster can be so accurate at predicting the future with the information available. High five, weather forecaster.

But, and this is a big "but," the future is not real—and that complicates things. I'll say it again. *The future is not real.* It is a construct. It is the end product of using our skills of pattern recognition and modeling. It can certainly seem real. We act like it is real. We react as if it is real. But it is not tangible. It is not real. For example, if a lion walked into your house (yikes), your danger response should go off. You should be having a panic attack. That is a real lion roaring in your foyer. But envisioning a lion showing up at your house because a lion got out of the zoo is not real. It is a construct. It is a thought. It is a concept. You have to be careful not to set off a panic attack at the *thought* of a lion. Make plans, lock the door, or get a gun. But you can do this without overwhelming fear; we will explore this more in a moment.

Like the weather forecaster, your predictions (based on your patterns and model) should not be set in stone. They can be and should be adjusted regularly. Like a weather forecaster, when information changes, you need to update your predictions. You need to update your view of your future.

This is important. Since the future is a construct, it can be changed. You can change the model, you can change the pattern, you can change the input information. Then, when you run the model into the future, your outcome will be different.

For many centuries, the prevailing construct was that the Earth was flat. Many observations formed the patterns that led to the concept of a flat Earth. And if the Earth is flat, then falling off the Earth is a possibility.

Let's imagine you are an Italian ship's captain in the 1400s. You sail out of port trying to find a quicker way to India and the vast riches that will be within reach with a shorter route. But you have a model that says the Earth is flat. If that construct is correct, you will eventually fall off the Earth. You have seen a waterfall before, so you know falling off the edge of the Earth will be worse—and will surely mean your death. Only a crazy person would take on the quest to find a shorter route on a flat Earth.

But the promise of wealth is calling you, so you decide to try. As you sail farther and farther from port, your fear increases. Your crew members are not as motivated as you, and their fear is starting to limit their desires. They want to turn back. Then you hit land. Unfortunately, it is not India, but it will still be an important discovery for the people back home. This journey has given you new information, and with it you start to make a new model of the Earth. In this new model, the Earth is not flat. It is round.

What? That is preposterous! But your experience has forced you to tweak your old model. If, as captain, your model changes from that of a flat Earth to a round Earth, then sailing around the world really is possible. You no longer face the possibility of falling off the earth. Instead, your challenge is one of logistics. That is quite a change.

No other organism on Earth possesses anything close to our ability to gather information, recognize patterns, make a model, and run it into the future. *Yeeeaaahhh humans!*

It is an incredible skill. We can look into the future and alter what we do now in order to change the future or, at least, to be better prepared for what will come. Ideally, you have been saving money for the day when you are old enough to retire. That means you have run a model that predicts that you will get old enough to retire and still be alive. You have taken money that you could spend now and put it in a place where you won't use it until you retire. But, like anything else, circumstances change, so you must continually monitor your situation and adjust your model. If you seek to retire well, the better your model, the more success you will have.

Even though the future is a construct and can be changed, we treat it as if it were real. It is so real that the future is now integrated into our everyday world. This is a new idea: ***The future is part of our environment.***

Our environment has been expanding for a hundred years. In the past, most people lived and died within their local community. The appearance of cars expanded humans' environment. Later, as airplanes became more common, our environment spread to cover the Earth. We can travel from one side of the world to the other in less than a day. Also, fortunately or unfortunately, the advent of the internet and the twenty-four-hour news cycle means events that happen on the other side of the Earth now affect us within hours.

So, we acknowledge that the human environment has expanded to encompass the whole globe. But what about the future? It still needs to be added to this lens through which we see our lives. It is not just what is happening in my building at this very moment that I care about, but also what will happen in a week or a year or a decade. Our view of the future feels tangible enough that we react as if it *were* real. And this is where the problems start to occur, because the future is *not* real. It is a construct. It is a prediction. It is a model of what we think will happen. But just as our environment has expanded to include the globe, so has it expanded to include the future.

> The second component of worry is focusing on the bad things that can happen.

All organisms, including humans, are wired to try to keep their environment safe. It is a primary part of staying alive and the reason we have a sensory system: to detect danger and dodge or destroy it. If you fail at this, you may end up dead. Organisms can miss good things and still survive, but if you fail to spot a danger, bad things happen. Let me give you an example. I have brought ten friends into your living room. Each has $10,000 that he or she is trying to give to you. In the corner is an eleventh person. This person has a machine gun trained on your head. Who in the room do you pay attention to?

Of course, you focus on the person with the machine gun. Although it would be nice to have the money, you have made it this far without an extra $10,000. Anyway, what good is $10,000 in your hand if you are shot dead? Your goal must be to dodge the danger, even if it means giving up a benefit.

You get the point. Humans are no different than other organisms when it comes to paying attention to danger in the immediate environment. But humans *are* different when you factor in the future. If the future is part of your environment, your natural instinct is to also keep an eye out for future threats. What does that mean? It means we tend to focus on the bad things that can happen in our future construct. This, in turn, feeds worry.

We are taking a primitive skill—keeping our environment safe—and applying it to the new environment that our mind skill has created, the future. This is an important survival mechanism for humans. We can identify potential dangers and take action to eliminate them or to protect ourselves if they do occur. If I envision the future and see a hurricane heading my way, I can reinforce my home or get the hell out of Dodge. If I know a dangerous person is lurking outside my house, I can call the police before I am hurt. In either case, I survive to face another day.

It is an incredible skill to be able to envision the future, spot potential threats, and stop them or protect ourselves before they happen. Unfortunately, not all humans have this skill. Newborns do not have the ability to envision the future. Infants have not crossed the threshold to mind yet. They cry when they are hungry, but do not envision the future and wonder what will happen if there is no money to buy formula. They simply cry and hope someone gives them something to eat. Patients with severe dementia are another group who are unable to scan the future for danger. They do not think, "How will I be taken care of in the future?" They just live for today.

Without the future, there is less to be afraid of in life. And that means there is no worry. If a surrounding environment is safe, people are happy. The adage that "Ignorance is bliss" is true. But so is the saying that "Knowledge is power." The infant and the severely demented patient cannot successfully navigate the world on their own because they lack the necessary skills. They need to be supervised by someone who does have the ability to envision the future.

In my practice, I have found that women tend to worry more than men. My theory is that men do worry, but they also minimize danger as a way to deal with their stress.

Trying not to stereotype, I think women's brains were adapted for the role of taking care of children. Looking into the future is a crucial skill if you are watching a toddler. A mother's ability to see danger and help her child avoid it will greatly increase her child's chances for survival. Men's brains, on the other hand, were designed to hunt for food, including woolly mammoths and other prey. This hunting was dangerous work. Focusing on everything that could go wrong would have kept primitive men from even attempting to kill a woolly mammoth, and that would have meant that their families went hungry. As men minimized the dangers they faced so that they could carry out essential tasks, they also lowered their level of worry.

My observation is by no means exclusive. There are plenty of worrying men and minimizing women. Interestingly, people on either end of this spectrum tend to be attracted to one another. A worrier likes to be around a minimizer. When the worrier is having a giant fear response, the minimizer is reassuring. When the minimizer is underreacting, the worrier takes the minimizer's head out of the clouds or removes their rose-colored glasses.

At first, this relationship works well. But, over time, it starts to fray. The worrier begins to mistrust the minimizer because of a couple of bad outcomes. Instead of being reassured, the worrier stops listening to the minimizer. The minimizer, meanwhile, hates to have every potential threat thrown onto the table; it makes it too hard to ignore the possibility of bad things happening. As the relationship deteriorates, the worrier cries, "Why do I have to do all the worrying?" while the minimizer is plopped in front of the TV, trying to ignore the worrier and everything being worried about. If you are a worrier, has this happened in your relationship?

There is something else that drives our worry: news media. We live in the middle of an Information Age, barraged by more information than we're able to process. As I noted before, knowledge is power. The more information you have, the more power you possess. But there is a side effect to this knowledge. The more we know, the more *bad outcomes* we are aware of. Interesting, isn't it? The smarter you are, the more negative outcomes you can imagine. Sometimes the smartest or the most well-informed person is also the biggest worrier.

Technology weaves into our worry in another way: it heightens how vivid threats can feel. With our technology, we have movies that seem wonderfully real. And often their story lines are built around catastrophic events. We sit in a theater chair and witness an asteroid striking Earth. Or maybe Earth is being destroyed by an alien race. Or humans are being killed by a virus or annihilated by a powerful warlord. Even entities that don't exist, like zombies or vampires, scare us in movies and make us worry about our future.

Movies aren't real, and most people can differentiate movies from reality. But there *are* real disasters and dramas (including your worst fear or nightmare) taking place around the world. Thanks to smartphones and twenty-four-hour news cycles, they are coming onto your radar in real time every day.

One point I want to be sure to make is that the rise of information is not just about the information. It is how it is being presented. It is the visual content that is particularly problematic. I call this the Video Effect. An example of the Video Effect is the story of a national football league player who received a 2-game suspension for punching his girlfriend. When the video was released, and people saw it with their own eyes, he never played football again. Eighty percent of the information that most humans take in is visual. Seeing is believing.

Indeed, we are far more reactive to what we see than what we hear or read. Reading a reporter's version of an army battle can be unsettling, but watching a video of people being shot and blown up is over-the-top distressing. And what are we being inundated with? Videos of every nightmarish occurrence the human mind can conjure up. It's no wonder stress and worry are at an all-time high.

Back to our immediate environment for a minute. My dog Ben's environment is what he can smell, hear, or see. For me, my environment is what I can smell, hear, or see—and the rest of the world. But it is even more than that. Science and computers can take us beyond our world to the rest of the universe—and that also means my environment now includes the future of all the universe. OMG! You can just imagine how many bad things I would have to be on alert for in an environment that size!

Our brains were programmed to watch for and respond to the bad things in our environment. But now, the range of our environment extends beyond our personal sensory system (what we can see, smell, hear, and so forth). Now it covers the entire planet and the universe and our future-looking projections for all of them! It's no wonder that the entire population of Earth is far more stressed today than in any other time of human existence. Stress levels among the general population are rising by the day, and the coping skills humans have developed are overwhelmed. This is making people more dysfunctional.

Being overwhelmed on its own is a stressor and one that we will deal with in a later chapter. As we examine worry, however, it is useful to know that worry is one of the components that leads to be people being overwhelmed.

I am sitting in front of my computer in 2020 during an event that explicitly captures everything I am talking about. In 2020, the COVID-19 virus pandemic is—literally—shutting down the world. The basis for the response to the pandemic is worry. People and governments are looking into the future, focusing on all the potential bad outcomes and sparking massive danger responses. People are exposed to minute-by-minute updates about the deadly virus. There are videos showing patients who are dying. The information is inescapable.

The antagonist is a virus that is invisible, contagious, incurable, and deadly. Or at least that is what news and social media sources are leading me to believe. In actuality, when considered in the context of other global infectious diseases, the coronavirus is not even among the Top Ten killers. Tuberculosis, malaria, and HIV, for example, are more common and more deadly. Still, with the extensive news coverage and the emphasis on worst-case scenarios by government officials (and experts who make their money by dreaming up worst-case scenarios), not only is the world shutting down temporarily, but humanity's fear is ramping up.

There has to be a better way to deal with this public-health challenge. In fact, I would bet that more damage is being caused by our attempts to control this virus than could ever be done by the virus itself. The pandemic story is the type of drama that leads to incalculable stress.

The third component of worry

We have examined two parts of worry—that we look into the future and, while doing that, we focus on bad things that can happen in our environment, which now includes the entire universe to the end of its existence. But it is the third component of worry that causes humans the most trouble. That is the danger response.

What is a danger response?

This topic is a whole book in itself, so I will give you a short version of the answer. When a human is put into an unknown situation or in a situation where death is a possible outcome, the body has two responses, fear or anger. These responses require no thinking; they occur so quickly that they seem automatic. These responses have been honed over millions of years to deal with situations in which you don't have time to think.

When you have a danger response, there are increases in cortisol and adrenaline in your body. There is constriction of your blood vessels. Blood is shunted away from your stomach to your muscles. Your heart rate ramps up. In less than a second, your body is ready to face a life-or-death scenario.

Sometimes fear is the predominant response. Fear brings two responses: freeze or flight. You are unable to react, or you run away. Circumstances and experience dictate which one occurs. If anger is the predominant response, you clench your teeth and your fists, and prepare for a fight. This response is meant to last until you get away or die. (Hopefully, you got away.)

In Robert Sapolsky's book *Why Zebras Don't Get Ulcers*, he addresses this with an example that also explains the book's title. A zebra smells or sees a lion, or maybe a neighboring zebra smells or sees a lion and makes that information known. The zebra doesn't waste time trying to figure out what level of danger there really is. The zebra takes off running. His body has responded with a fear response, and it has called on every physiological reserve to get the animal out of there as fast as possible. However, after a few minutes, the fear response stops. The zebra can no longer see or smell a lion, his body calms down, and he goes back to eating grass until he senses some other danger.

In a similar vein, a gorilla might be confronted with another, unfamiliar gorilla. His response is to get ready for a fight. That is what anger is designed for. Within seconds, the gorilla's body goes through changes that make him ready to use his muscles, reduce bleeding, constrict blood vessels in the skin, and so forth. The fight won't last long. Either one will die, or one or both will withdraw. Either way, the anger response goes away, and, when it does, the gorilla that is still standing goes back to eating leaves.

Humans' danger response is similar to that of other animals—with one decisive difference. Humans have a concept of the future, and they have constructs related to that future. A zebra shuts off his fear response when there is no more detectable danger in his environment. But humans can continue to have a danger response. Humans can envision the future and worry that a lion will return. What if their back pain flared when they were trying to run away from the lion? What if their child was in the yard when a lion appeared? What if the danger was not a lion but an assailant, and that assailant came back with a knife or a gun? A human's danger response keeps going. Since it is not tied to the reality of the environment, there is nothing to make it stop.

In the book *The Worry Trick*, author David Carbonell calls this "What If?" thinking. What if the lion comes back? The "what if" just as easily elicits a danger response as a lion standing in front of you. You can "what if" yourself for days and weeks and years, propelling yourself with fear and anger—and nothing will stop it, either, since the danger isn't real. The danger is only a thought in your head.

Your danger response was designed to go on for only a short period of time. That means a chronic danger response causes a lot of wear and tear on your body. The chronic surges of cortisol and adrenaline lead to sleep problems, immune deficiency, skin rashes, ulcers, heart attacks, pain, and other physical effects. This is another reason why humans are struggling so much these days.

If you envision only the future and focus only on bad outcomes, you will be depressed but healthy. It is when you have a physiological danger response and *it doesn't stop* that you get in trouble.

Let's look at an example. Scientists have predicted the sun will explode in four billion years (give or take a day or two). That is an interesting tidbit of information. Scientists arrived at that prediction by making a model of how a star works, how big the sun is, and running the model into the future. The sun exploding would be a bad thing for humans. Our planet would either explode or become so cold that nothing would survive.

I can think about all that and not really react. It is only when I add worry and my danger response to the equation that the information turns into something bad to deal with.

I don't want to feel fear. My physiological arousal of fear makes me feel bad. It makes me want to hide or run away. It is an unpleasant sensation, and I am willing to do a lot of things to make fear stop. I want to be happy and feel pleasant and blissful. I want to be in my Happy Place. But fear gets in the way of that. This is the most uncomfortable part of worry.

If I simply ponder what will happen when the sun explodes in 4 billion years, I am playing a mind game. It's when I add fear that it becomes a matter of life and death. Fear keeps me awake at night; it makes me edgy and short with people around me. It makes me feel desperate and changes the thresholds of what I am willing to do. Most people can manage the fear of the sun blowing up but not everyone. And what if I step it up and use, instead of the exploding sun, an example like a terrorist on a plane I am taking? This might occur to me because a plane was blown up in Malaysia yesterday. Now my fear is jacked up. Now I can't think. I can't sleep. I have to do something to alleviate this feeling, but there is nothing to stop the fear because what I am afraid of hasn't happened. It is in the future. In a *theoretical* future. It isn't real, but it sure as heck *feels* real. My dog, Ben, is incapable of this reaction. His sensory system would say, "Everything is fine. Let's get on the plane and go." I am jumping out of my skin worrying there is a terrorist who might blow up my plane. Maybe I would even stay in my car because I decided today is not a good day to fly.

Please tell me you're going to show me how can I stop worrying. That's why I'm here.

I am going to start with a straightforward truth. You can't stop worrying. In fact, I don't want you to stop worrying. Worry is important to your survival. The inability to worry is like the failure to feel pain. It *sounds* good, but when burn your hand on a stove and don't know it because there is no pain sensation, you realize that pain is part of your safety toolkit. The ability to feel pain is a survival skill. In the same way, you need worry because it helps you avoid the bad things in life.

But what is happening right now is that you don't need as *much* of the worry as you have. What you need is to learn how to worry efficiently.

When you worry efficiently, you get the benefits of looking into the future without the side effects. You want to get the benefits of looking into the future, monitoring for bad things, but with fewer and shorter danger responses. The rest of this chapter tells you how to rebalance your response.

How do I do that?

The answer lies in the definitions and concepts we went through earlier this chapter.

First, you must realize the future is a construct. It hasn't happened. When you begin to think of the future as only a made-up theory of what will (or could) happen, it is easier to cut back your reaction.

Second, give thanks that you can envision the future. Not every human can say this. Infants and brain-damaged humans don't have the ability to envision the future. The fact that you bought this book to help you have a better, less-stressed life tells me you are smart enough to envision a future. It is a skill that humans are the world champion at. No other organism on Earth comes even close to our skill of looking into the future. How cool is that? Celebrate it.

Third, when you're looking into the future, there are two possible paths. Bad things can happen, or good things can happen. Your brain has been set up to focus on the bad things. But you have the ability to choose. You can focus on the good things that might happen. When you focus on the bad things, you feel bad. But here is an interesting truth: When you focus on the good things, you feel good. How simple is that?

Actually, it sounds simple, but it is not easy to do. Your brain has been wired to concentrate on bad things. Even if that were not true, you probably have trained yourself for years to focus on the bad things. Like the patient in my office last week: She told me how much she worries. I asked her what she worries about, and she had an impressively extensive list of things that came immediately to mind with barely any effort or thought. Then I asked what good things could happen in the future. It was as if no one had ever asked her that question. She had to think long and hard, and she barely came up with more than a couple things that might qualify as good outcomes. She quickly swamped these with more likely events that would prevent the good things from happening.

Focusing on bad things is a habit. It is like smoking. You can stop for a while, but the habit often drags you back. People can stop worrying for a while, but the habit drags them back.

I'm here to say that you can worry less. It will require practice and desire. I know you can do it if you follow these guidelines. First, when you envision the future, I want you to make a list of the bad things that can happen as well as the good things that can happen. Your habit has been to do the first and not the second, so it will be challenging at the beginning. Secondly, I want you to focus on the good things happening. That will give you a good feeling.

Let's use an example. You decide you want to write an autobiography. You sit down in front of the computer or the notepad or the typewriter. You envision the future and realize it is unlikely you will ever get this book written. This makes you sad. Feeling sad that the book will never be written, you start to cry. You close the computer and decide writing a book wasn't such a good idea anyway.

Now let's start over. You sit down to write your autobiography, and you think it will never be written, but you also think, "What if it *does* get written?" You imagine yourself on TV, being interviewed by a TV show host and talking about your life and your struggles writing the book. Thanks to your success as an author, you open your checkbook and find more money than has ever been in your account before. Your friends and family think more highly of you because your book is a success, and you got to meet the TV show host in person. How does that feel? Good, right?

There is a key term connected to the process of worrying more efficiently. It is **Realistic Optimism**. This refers to looking into the future and focusing on the good things that can happen. Doing so will make you feel good and give you the energy to continue focusing on the positive. Realistic optimism will counteract the negative feelings that come when you keep your attention on the bad things that can happen.

Optimism is a hopefulness about the future, a confidence that good things will happen. But you *can't* just jump from worry to optimism. After all, you worry for a reason. You don't want to ignore or underestimate a bad thing that could occur. That's where the *realism* part of the phrase comes in. You can't live with only rose-colored glasses. You do need to acknowledge that bad things can and do happen—and you need to prepare for them. But you don't have to *focus* on them. After all, the future is neither real nor reliably predictable. By focusing on the good things and, consequently, feeling good, you will be a much happier person, and you will have more energy to deal with life as it comes along.

Realistic optimism allows you to be prepared for a bad outcome but without all the negative feelings that are consuming you now. Let's pretend again that you are writing a book. Life with realistic optimism enables you to sit down and write. You'll have the energy you need, and you will be way more likely to finish your manuscript. *Yeaahhhhh!*

Let's use another example to illustrate how this plays out. You get a notice from the IRS on the same day your cousin gets a notice from the IRS. You are both being audited. Yikes. You both think right away that this will end badly. You will have to pay your accountant, you will owe the IRS money, and you could end up in jail. But you have read this book, and, because of that, you understand realistic optimism. You call your accountant to prepare your defense, but you focus on an outcome in which you will not owe the IRS money and you will not end up in jail. This is a much more pleasant scenario and makes you feel good. You can even think that maybe the IRS will owe you money. *Ha!* You sleep well. You might even walk around with a smirk on your face, imagining how much the IRS owes you.

Your cousin has not read this book. (You should give your cousin this book as a birthday or Christmas gift!) Your cousin thinks about his IRS notice and spends the next year fearing that he will lose everything. His fear keeps him up at night. He starts drinking alcohol to squelch the never-ending worry that has gripped his life. He is losing his hair. He is miserable.

After a yearlong audit, the IRS verdict arrives in a thick envelope. You and your cousin both owe the IRS money. You are both unhappy. But you have had a year of sleep while thinking that things would work out—and you prepared just in case they didn't. You have the energy to deal with this setback. Your cousin, however, is devastated. He is exhausted, bedraggled, inebriated, and suffering from hair loss. He has no energy to deal with this new crisis. He makes bad choices and ends up in more trouble.

Oh, wait—there's more news. It turns out the IRS made a mistake, and you both get a $5,000 refund. You had focused on this outcome, so you feel vindicated and happy and wonder where you will use the newfound windfall. Your cousin is so exhausted he can barely register what just happened. Even though the outcome is good, he has been miserable for a year—hardly worth it for $5,000.

See the difference? Neither of you knew a year ago what the envelope would have in it. So why not focus on a good outcome? Yes, you need to be realistic, call your accountant, send in the required paperwork, follow up on deadlines, and ask your friends for advice—but keep your focus on the good outcome. This will make you feel better and give you more energy in the event something bad does happen.

It will take practice. It is not automatic yet. You will have to overcome a habit you have honed over your lifetime, but I know you can get there.

How do I do that?

I told you to think up a list of good things and bad things that could occur. But, do you remember that I also said I want to teach you to be more efficient? To that end, I want you to write down your list. Writing it down is important for efficiency. Your written list has several advantages:

1. Ink is better than think. Ink is indelible and permanent. Thinking is an amazing skill, but it requires energy and memory. You may be prone to forgetting. You may find yourself going over the same thought again and again. **Write it down.**

2. It takes more energy to write than to think, so writing down your outcomes makes you focus. It makes you direct your thoughts more precisely so that you can reduce how much you have to write.

3. Writing it down becomes a habit. And having a new habit will help break the old one. Practice this new habit of writing until it becomes automatic.

4. Writing frees up your mind. You can focus all your mind on the list, instead of half on the list and half on remembering the list.

5. You only have to do it once. Once it is written, you don't have to keep remembering. Most people review a mental list over and over again. They are afraid they will forget the bad outcomes—and they probably will—so they think and rethink the bad consequence. This brings on a danger response. As my good friend Hal says, "The palest ink is better than the best memory." Write it down, and you don't have to remember anymore.

6. When you wake up in the middle of the night worrying, you can relax because you already have everything written down. Unless you have something new to add, you can feel reassured—and go back to sleep.

7. Problem-solving is much easier when you see the problem in front of you, rather than having to think about it. It is more work up front, but you save yourself from repeated loops of worry.

8. You can share your thoughts with friends and professionals. And that allows them to have a better idea of what you are thinking. They can read your notes more easily than they can read your mind. Even more, they can offer their own insights.

9. Because I said so. (LOL—that was my Dad channeling through me.)

For the bad things on your list, you can eventually begin to fashion protections against what you fear or figure out ways to change the present to avoid the bad outcome. But your real focus needs to be on the good list and feeling good *now*.

I want to bring back the example of my patient who was worrying about breast cancer. Her case is a good illustration of another tool to reduce worry. I call it the **Worry Organizer**. I have been using this worry sheet for years, and it works.

I had my patient, Mary, fill out a worry sheet. The first category is "What am I worried about?" In her case, the obvious answer was that she was worried about getting breast cancer. In her mind, this was not unreasonable, given her family history. The idea of a breast-cancer diagnosis generated a huge fear response because she knew all the things that could come along with that disease and its prognosis.

Although Mary barely needed to think about what to put in the first category, "What am I worried about?" it is not always clear for all people. Sometimes the obvious answer, like breast cancer, is not the only or even the primary worry. Going through chemotherapy may be more of a worry than breast cancer itself. Don't rush through this category. Sometimes what you are worried about is only the superficial issue, and there is more going on. Maybe you are worried about going to an event, but, upon more reflection, what you are really worried about is facing an estranged lover. Take some time to think about what seems to be your main worry, keeping in mind there might be other or imbedded worries.

Less Stress Doc	**Worry Organizer**		www.thelessstressdoc.com	
What am I worried about?	Why am I worried about that?	How likely or dangerous is this?	What can I do about this?	What if the worst happens?

The second category on the worry sheet asks, "Why am I worried?" For Mary, a family history of breast cancer means her chance of having breast cancer is higher. Also, she has seen other family members deal with cancer treatments, and she knows how devastating they can be.

You might need to spend some time on this category. It might take some exploration. If you are worried about seeing a friend, it may be because you will have to travel over a bridge and you have a phobia about bridges. Seeing the friend is not the worry—going over the bridge is. Sometimes self-esteem is an underlying component to why you are worried. You are worried that you won't live up to expectations.

The third category focuses on how likely it is that the thing causing your worry will really happen—and how dangerous it is if it does happen. I always think of this as the most controversial category. This is the category that leads to most fights, even though it should be the most objective. Mary felt like breast cancer was at least a 90 percent likelihood. She figured that, with a strong family history, 90 percent might even be an underestimate. When she was asked how dangerous it would be if she had breast cancer, she said there was a 90 percent likelihood she would die. With these kinds of estimates, no wonder she was worried. She had essentially given herself a death sentence. All her dreams were gone. Her family would be without a wife, mother, sister, or daughter. Why even go on if these dreadful statistics are looming over her? Mary lived her life drenched in the desperation that comes to someone who knows they are going to die.

But here is the elegance to this category on the worry list: It is the most objective category, the most measurable, the one based on numbers and percentages. In Mary's situation, there is data, and here's what I was able to tell her: Your chance of getting breast cancer is 15 percent, and your chance of dying from breast cancer is 15 percent. Mary looked at me in disbelief. I had to show her the medical articles, but she finally was able to process this information and change her outlook. Once she was willing to believe these numbers, a smile took over her face.

She said that 15 percent is *so small*. Her life was given back to her. All that worry was no longer necessary.

Fortunately for Mary, there were proven numbers to use. In many cases, this is not true. Take the circumstance in which parents are discussing/arguing with their teenager about attending a concert. The conversation starts with the parents worried that their child will get in trouble at the event. The chances are small but real. As long as the parents are nearby, they figure, they will be able to gain control of the situation if trouble surfaces. Of course, the teenager thinks the chance of getting in trouble is minuscule—so small, in fact, that it is not worth discussing how to handle a problem if it should occur.

Now let's add a wrinkle. The concert is in an adjacent state. The probability of trouble has not really changed much, but the parents' perception of danger has gone up dramatically. The parents will not be able to easily fix or gain control if a problem occurs in another state. Their tentative "Yes" answer about going to the concert turns into a definite "No." The teenager still thinks the chance of a problem is so small that whether a problem occurs in-state or out-of-state should have no bearing on the decision. This parent-teen discussion is headed toward a fight. It will escalate into name-calling, punishments, hurt feelings, and bruised egos.

This is where statistics come in. With statistics, you can at least try to have a civil, less-emotional discussion. The numbers give you a chance to add rationality to your arguments. If the parent says the chances of a problem are 10 percent, the teenager can counter that they are 1 percent. Perhaps the police even have public statistics on how likely this problem is. If not, at least the parents and teen can meet halfway, compromising on a 5 percent probability. And then the discussion can focus on what to do if a problem does occur, taken in the context of a more concrete idea of what the dangers are and how to resolve them.

The next column in the Worry Organizer looks at how to avoid the problem. If you are Mary, you can get regular mammograms and do breast self-exams. You can get a genetic test. This category, in effect, helps you come up with a to-do list. This has several benefits. It forces you to think about the problem in a focused manner and then write it down. If, over time, you think of new solutions, you can add them to the list. This list also becomes something you can show to family, friends, or professionals to get their input.

I was able to tell Mary the things she could do to decrease her chances of getting breast cancer, including diet, supplements, and genetic testing. For the case of the parents and their teenager, the parents could talk to other parents whose child wants to go to the same concert or who has attended other concerts. They could talk to their local police officer to gets his/her input into ways to keep their child safe.

The last column in the Worry Organizer is the emergency backup plan if the problem occurs. Mary can make a list of breast-cancer centers. She can investigate online. She can put proposed plans for getting medical care into place. She can have contingency plans for work and family. She can make a will. She may never need any of these things, but I find that people have less worry when they have an emergency plan in place. It's one less thing to think about when it is late at night and worry/danger response starts. For the parents and teenager, the backup plan might mean having AAA or making sure they have the phone number of a good lawyer. These contingency plans will force a discussion on possible outcomes and their solutions before they occur. It is better to be prepared than to be sorry.

And again, remember that, when the plans are written down, they have to be done only once. The next time the concert question comes up, the discussion has already been explored and written down. Remember, I am trying to show you how to *worry efficiently.*

What else can be done to alleviate my worry?

Since worry is really a danger response, there are two main ways to alleviate the physiological reaction to it. You can give the fear somewhere to go. Exercise will give your adrenaline an outlet. When you are physically tired, it is more difficult to feel fear. You don't have the energy. When you are exercising, your brain is engaged in the task at hand and cannot wander as easily to "What if?" If you exercise alone, you can enjoy the solitude. If you exercise in a group, you can enjoy the bonding that occurs when you engage with other humans in a similar pursuit. Either way, pleasure is stimulated, and your worry and stress diminish.

You can also do the opposite. You can engage in a relaxation technique or meditate. There is a physiological reason relaxation and meditation work. They increase the parasympathetic response (opposite of adrenaline) in your body. This is the inverse of fear. The more parasympathetic stimulation, the less sympathetic stimulation. Relaxation and meditation reduce your fear by pushing the balance toward relaxation and away from a fear response.

These techniques are very effective, but it has been my experience that patients have to practice before they grow proficient at them. The first time you try a relaxation exercise might not be very relaxing. Keep at it. The more practice, the better it will work. You can get so good that just *thinking* about the relaxation technique will start to relax you and reduce your fear.

There are two relaxation techniques I especially like to use. The first is something I learned in an acting class in college. (My backup plan if I didn't get into medical school was to be an actor on the TV series *General Hospital*.) I lie in a comfortable position. I take slow, deep breaths. Inhalation is 1/3, exhalation is 2/3. I focus on the air coming in and going out. After I get into a rhythm, I visualize energy and stress leaving my body through my fingers and toes. My muscles become heavy. They become so heavy and relaxed that I can't pick them up. Once my arms and legs are relaxed, I focus on my facial muscles. I imagine the tension leaving and feel like my face is drooping. I continue to focus on my breathing and the sensation of how heavy and relaxed my body is. When I am done with relaxing, I reluctantly come back and sit up. My balance has been reset, and I feel better.

The second technique I use is *guided imagery*. I start with the first technique and get relaxed. Then I pick my safe place. I open a door, and I'm at a beach. I see the ocean and the sun. I smell the suntan lotion and food being grilled. I feel waves lap at my feet and taste the saltwater. The heat of the sun warms my skin. The more senses involved, the better guided imagery works. I can spend as long as I like at the beach (and not get sunburned). When I am done, I get up and walk through the doorway in my mind—and close it behind me. I'm back in the real world, but I feel more relaxed. You can pick your own safe place. It needs to be somewhere you can feel relaxed and comfortable.

As a doctor, I also add the category of medication as a way to address worry. Some people have such a potent fear reaction and, consequently, such overwhelming worry, that my earlier suggestions and techniques are not effective enough. These people's lives are miserable and dysfunctional. There are several medicines that can be prescribed. These are always used in conjunction with the other modalities I have talked about. The broad categories are antidepressants such as Zoloft or other SSRIs, benzodiazepams like Ativan or Klonipin, B-blockers like Inderal; the latest include neuroleptics such as Gabapentin and antipsychotics such as Seroquel. These need to be discussed on an individual basis with someone who knows you. (They are beyond the scope of this book.) Call me or your own doctor for more individual advice about this alternative.

One final thing I wanted to discuss is hypnosis, coupled with Neurolinguistic Programming (NLP). I have become certified in hypnosis with neurolinguistic programming. After learning the technique and seeing how effective it can be, I wished I had learned it sooner and had more time to work with patients. Let me start with what hypnosis is *not*. It is not putting people in a trance and making them bark like a dog. When you are under hypnosis, you will always be aware of what is going on, and you can always stop it. You are in control. Always.

Hypnosis allows you to relax but in a focused way. It allows you access to more information stored in your brain by tuning out the noise that surrounds you. It gives you more conscious control of what is going on in your brain. While you are relaxed with hypnosis, there are a variety of techniques that NLP offers to eliminate phobias, halt addictions, reframe past traumas, and so on. You can do hypnosis on your own, but the Neurolinguistic Programming requires someone who is trained to work with you.

I have a patient who was beaten up at work. She thought she was going to die. She survived the assault, but every time her memory of this event was triggered, she had a panic attack. She had 20 years of panic. Psychotherapy, medications, alcohol, church . . . none alleviated the devastating panic attacks. We decided to try hypnosis with NLP. During our session, she reimagined the scene but with a lot of safety measures in place. She remembered being hit and then passing out. When she woke up, she saw that the assailant was punching a co-worker. She was convinced he was going to kill the co-worker. She had a choice. She could pretend to be unconscious or try to help her co-worker. She chose to help the co-worker. She got up and phoned for help. She distracted the assailant. She and her co-worker were rescued.

When she came out of hypnosis, I was astounded at what she had accomplished. I told her she was a hero. She risked her own life to help someone else. She had forgotten that part of the incident. Her memory had been as a victim and was cloaked in pain, fear, a sense of things being out of control. By reframing her memory, she was a hero, and she left my office with a smile on her face. Before our session, the mere mention of the incident would spark a physical reaction of fear. After our session, she would calmly describe what happened—without fear or a sense of victimization. Her psychologist noticed the change in her and asked what had happened. She had reframed her memory.

There is a second part to this story. Two weeks later, the same patient called and asked for another NLP session. In reframing the memory of her assailant, she had uncovered another deeply hidden trauma. When she was eight, her father had been drunk, and he cut her mother with a knife. Her memory was of blood and fear and isolation and having to take care of her mother by herself. Under hypnosis, her memory was more accurate, and she recalled that her brother had been there, too. She had tried to shield him. Then she remembered a neighbor had come by and taken the two children next door while the paramedics attended to her mother. Again, her memory had been reframed. She was more concerned with taking care of her brother than herself. And she realized her neighborhood had a close-knit group of people who helped each other. She was not alone.

This patient cried with relief. She has been a different person since our two sessions. She is more at peace with herself. She has cut back on medications. She now helps other people (of course) in a hospice program. I wish everyone could so effectively reframe their trauma.

Now that you have read this chapter and understand worry, let me know if you can think up any techniques for worrying less. Give me your suggestions on my website: TheLessStressDoc.com

LET'S RECAP
Definition of Worry
Worry is using your mind skill of looking into the future, focusing on the bad things that could happen, and having a fear/danger response in the present.

Human Skills: Envisioning the future
Side Effects: Fear
Tools:

- Worry efficiently, don't eliminate worry entirely.

- Realistic Optimism-looking into the future and acknowledging bad things can happen but focusing on good outcomes. This leads to a pleasant physiological response and allows you to prepare yourself in case something bad does happen.

- Worry Organizer-this exercise makes you think about the real cause of your worry, how likely or dangerous it is that your fear will come true, and how you can avoid the problem or design an emergency backup plan if it does happen.

- Exercise

- Relaxation techniques reduce fear by counteracting the physiological reaction.

- Medications can be used under a doctor's supervision.

- Hypnosis with NLP can be an effective technique.

- Contact me for more individual advice at TheLessStressDoc .com

- You can get more information about NLP from the book NLP: The Essential Guide to Neurolinguistic Programming or contacting the authors, Tom Hoobyar, Tom Dotz, or Susan Sanders.

Hopefully this chapter will have reduced your worry and your fear response, and the worry that you continue to have will be more efficient. You should end up with more energy to devote to solving your problems and more time in your Happy Place, content and happy as you anticipate good things to come.

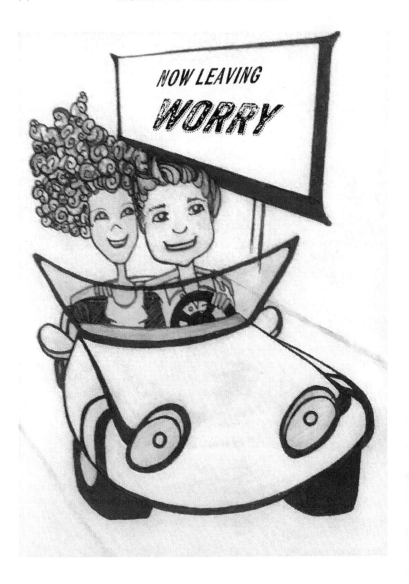

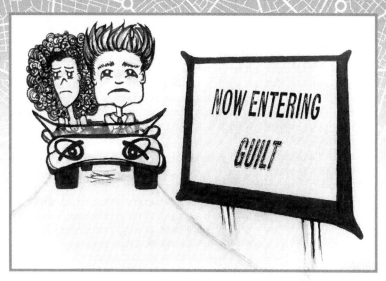

CHAPTER THREE

Guilt

Are You Beating Yourself Up With Guilt?

In this chapter I will define guilt. I will tell you about Maryanne. I will show the difference between guilt and shame. I will define the concept of what an emotion is. I will define right and wrong. Then I will show you how to have less guilt, by understanding what group you're in, who the judge is, what the rules are, and what the goal of your group is. Next, I will show you the process of forgiveness for others and for yourself. I will touch on cognitive behavioral therapy, hypnosis, NLP, and medication.

Definition of Guilt: Guilt is what occurs when the negative emotion from the brain known as "shame" is combined with the mind's ability to label actions and ideas as right or wrong.

Ok, here goes. I told you I am willing to share my story with patients. Many doctors keep a wall between their personal life and their professional life. I am not one of those doctors. If you are going to share with me, I have to be willing to share with you. Here is the story of mine that illustrates guilt.

Maryanne came to my office as a regular patient. I had been in practice a few years, so I was new but not totally naïve. She had been having problems with indigestion, and I had prescribed medication and diet to alleviate her symptoms. She came to my office one day with chest pain. She was not nauseated, and she was not having crushing substernal chest pain. She was not sweaty or having pain going down her arm. I examined her heart and lungs, and did an EKG. It was normal. I came to the conclusion that the medicine I had given her for her indigestion wasn't working as well as I was hoping. So, I adjusted her medication and sent her home to be rechecked in a couple of weeks. Since I am sharing this story, you can guess where this went.

That night, Maryanne was taken to the hospital and diagnosed with a heart attack. It was a bad heart attack. She survived my mistake, but her heart was irreparably damaged. Her heart was pumping at 25% of where it should be. I was a devastated young physician. How could I have been so wrong?

Making matters worse for me, Maryanne stayed with me as a patient. She did not blame me or hold me responsible for her heart attack. She still trusted me to give her sound medical advice. I saw her monthly because her medications had to be adjusted to keep her functioning with her weakened heart. Every time I saw Maryanne, I would be distraught. Not outwardly, but inside, I knew her life had been altered because of my failure to diagnose her heart attack at that first visit. She would confide in me that she liked her windows clean, but, after cleaning only one window, she would have to rest for two days to get her energy back. I tried my hardest to be conscientious with her care and do everything I could to make her life as comfortable and as functional as I could. But I had that same guilt reaction every time she came into my office.

As I am writing this, I am getting tears in my eyes. It was more than 30 years ago. I am still feeling some guilt, but here is the key: The next day, I had to see a different patient with chest pain. And the next week, another patient with chest pain. It would be foolish to just send every patient to the hospital. I had to corral my guilt and go through the workup each time and make a decision about the patient in my office. I had to learn to keep my guilt and shame out of my decision-making process (as much as possible) with the next patient. It was a difficult lesson, but I had to find a way to still function as a doctor after a decision I made was the wrong one and cost my patient her health.

I didn't learn all at once. I didn't have my book at the time. But, now, after reading, exploring, and analyzing, I have found a way to minimize my guilt so that I could help the thousands of patients I saw after Maryanne. My experience with Maryanne made me a better doctor. It made me take more time with each decision, now knowing every decision I make could negatively affect a patient's life. I had lost that cavalier attitude that comes with youth and ignorance.

Maryanne never used the words "I forgive you." But she kept coming as a patient, so, clearly, she had forgiven me. I had to learn to forgive myself. In the rest of the chapter, I will go through what guilt is and then how to reduce it, so that you, too, can function in a better way.

The first step to dealing with any problem is to define it. When I ask people what guilt is, I usually get the answer that it is doing something wrong. I would agree with this definition, but, as you will see in the next chapter about regret, it has to be differentiated from making a bad choice.

There is something else about guilt that you need to know. It is intrinsically linked to the emotion of shame.

What is shame?

Shame is what I call a *primary emotion*. Some of the other primary emotions are fear, anger, pleasure, happiness, sadness, hunger, curiosity, lust, and bonding. These are emotions we are born knowing. We don't have to learn them. No one taught me how to be afraid or how to feel lust or how to be curious. What I did have to learn, however, is what to be afraid of or the reasons to get angry.

Primary emotions come from the brain. We are not the only organism with primary emotions. My dog will exhibit shame. Elephants show signs of sadness when a member of the herd dies. Other animals also have primary emotions.

But I want to go deeper than shame. I want to ask the question, "What is an emotion?" This is another one of those words we use and understand, but when someone asks for a definition, we are at a loss. You can use "emotion" in a sentence. You can name several emotions. But defining the word is more challenging. I will tell you that I have asked professionals, and they have the same problem. The dictionary defines an emotion as a feeling, and, of course, the definition of feeling is an emotion.

Here is the definition that works for me. **An emotion is a coordinated neurohormonal pattern that is set off by a push-button, preprogrammed trigger.**

Got that? I'll explain in more detail.

| The first part of my definition of "emotion" is the neurohormonal response.

Emotions emerge from a pattern of hormones being released—hormones such as cortisol, adrenaline, or oxytocin—and a neurological pattern that triggers muscles, blood vessels, heart rate, and other functions. This pattern is recognizable. I can tell when you are angry or when you are afraid. When your fists are clenched and your teeth are bared, I don't think you are lusting after someone. When you are hiding in the corner and your heart rate is 120, I don't think you are exhibiting curiosity. We label the pattern with words like *fear, lust, anger, curiosity*. Each emotion has a different neurohormonal pattern. There is, obviously, some overlap, and people can experience more than one emotion at the same time. It turns out that emotions are very hard to study, because our mind modifies our reaction, and our learned experiences can lead to very different reactions. If I see blood, I will be curious about where it came from. Other people may react with fear or disgust. Same stimulus, totally different reaction.

| The second part of the definition is that an emotion is set off by a trigger.

A trigger is something in the environment that sets off the coordinated neurohormonal response. The trigger can be external, like a gunshot or a beautiful painting. Or it can be internal. Maybe you are thinking about when you got married or had your first child, and that will trigger an emotional response. There is debate about how triggers get attached to the neurohormonal response. It could be you were born with the connection. Or it could be you acquired the connection through learning. Either way, there is an anatomical connection between the trigger and the emotional response that occurs over time and gets strengthened with repetition.

It is preprogrammed.

It is in the wiring of my brain. It does not require thinking or problem-solving. The connection has been set up and is waiting to kick in. The fear reaction or the anger reaction or the lust reaction has an anatomical connection. Thinking is slow compared to these connections.

It is push-button.

The trigger hits a button in the brain, and the button sets off the reaction. The important thing to know is that a single trigger will set off a specific emotion—and very quickly. A grizzly bear in my tent triggers a fear emotion in milliseconds.

To recap, an emotion is a coordinated pattern or response that involves hormones and nerves. Each emotion has a specific pattern. It is set off by a trigger that can be innate or learned. It becomes hard-wired or an anatomical tract that no longer requires thinking or problem-solving. The trigger pushes an anatomical button that gets the pattern started. It is designed to be very fast, and it was set up to ensure our survival. In an unfamiliar situation, I rely on my emotions to get me through until I have time to learn what to do the next time.

Shame is one of these emotions. Humans and animals have a shame response. I don't teach my dog how to be ashamed, but I do teach him what to be ashamed about. Same for my children. Same for me. Same for you.

If that is shame, where does guilt fit in?

Guilt is a secondary emotion—one that works off a primary emotion—like fear, shame, anger, or lust—and then adds a separate component that comes from the mind. Remember Stratasphere? The inner layer is the primary emotion. This we share with other animals that have a brain. To the inner layer of shame, humans have added a new layer that is guilt. It is the side effect of the emergent property that comes from a mind—it reacts to the concept of right and wrong.

When shame is the primary emotion, the mind must establish ideas around right and wrong for guilt to appear. Other animals do not have the concepts of right and wrong. They can be trained to do a task or to stop a behavior with positive or negative feedback, but that is not the same as understanding right and wrong. If my dog Ben tries to eat from my dinner plate, I sternly tell him to stop. He understands the negative feedback and will respond as ashamed, but he doesn't understand that his behavior is wrong. He only understands he shouldn't do it. Shame in animals comes from the negative feedback that helps shape behavior in an animal group. I doubt alligators have shame, but apes and dogs definitely have it.

Humans have taken shame to a higher level. You'll recall that we have a mind skill that other animals don't have. We have concepts, ideas. Because of that, we can train a human to have a shame reaction to a thought. If you are so mad at your friend that you want to hurt them, you should feel shame. In an ever-enlarging group of humans, we need an agreed-upon set of rules to maintain safety and cooperation. We also need a way to enforce those rules. So, shame becomes guilt at the mind level.

Right and wrong are interesting concepts. I have spent some time exploring what right and wrong mean. What I learned is that right and wrong must be defined by the group, and each group has its own definition. What is right in one group may be diametrically opposed to what is right in another group. I am a member of the American Medical Association. I would not go to a meeting in Chicago and bring a gun to kill people. That would be wrong. But if I were a member of SEAL Team 6, I might travel with multiple weapons and kill anyone necessary to complete my mission. As a SEAL, I would be rewarded with a Medal of Honor for doing that. But if I did that as a doctor at a medical meeting in Chicago, I would be put in jail for the rest of my life. Right and wrong are defined by the group with which we are affiliated at the time.

What about the rules? Sometimes the rules are written down, as they are in the huge book specifying baseball rules or in the shelves of law books for a country. Sometimes they are agreed upon but not written. What a teenager considers fashionable is not written down. However, a teenager doesn't want to violate the fashion rules of his or her circle. The punishment would be, at best, teasing. Sometimes people break rules not by choice but because they don't know the rules. I was once at a meeting where a colleague had been violating a national law. But he had no idea of his breach until a government official pulled him aside after the meeting to explain the transgression. Fortunately, my colleague did not go to jail, and he quickly corrected his ways. Knowing the rules is important when determining right and wrong.

Rules do not exist in a void. Rather, they hinge on goals. "Thou shalt not kill" as a rule doesn't always work. If you are in a war, killing becomes the norm and the means to survive. It becomes the measure of who wins, which, consequently, determines who was right. When it comes to rules, the goals are critical. The government takes money from your paycheck. If your boss took money from your paycheck to pay for his boat, you would be mad. (Plus, your boss would be breaking the rules.) But if the government takes your money to pay for a boat that will defend you (and others) against a deadly enemy, you are happy to have your money taken because it ensures your safety. The goal is important.

To operate this system of rules and goals, you also need judges. The judge is there to interpret close calls or resolve outright disputes. Judges come in many forms. There are the judges with a robe and gavel. But a judge could just as easily be a teenager who determines the current fashion statement. It could be a referee on the field of play or a replay official in another city with access to a camera feed. It could be an election official who verifies the vote of people by their ballots. It could be a Supreme Being or God. The judge takes into consideration the group, the current definition of its rules, and the goal of the rules, in order to come to a decision. The group has given the judge the authority to issue the final judgment of right and wrong. The judge is powerful within the group, which is why a judge's role must be as unbiased as possible.

We can see the benefit of right and wrong if a group is to live harmoniously. Without right and wrong, we end up with anarchy, which is not a productive state. Nevertheless, right and wrong can lead to conflict. A young Hindu man falls in love with an older American woman who is Catholic. Isn't that wrong on many levels? But what about love being blind—plus, don't rules change? If you are following yesterday's rules rather than the changed rules of today, you are in the position of breaking the rules—even though your very same behavior was exemplary yesterday. I have had a personal experience with this. When I started my medical practice, I recognized that patients suffering chronic pain were being underserved. Over the next 15 years, the medical establishment taught me that we were undertreating patients in pain, and we would be punished if we didn't do a better job. Then for the next 15 years, the same medical establishment taught me that we were causing an opioid epidemic, and we would be punished for writing prescriptions for pain meds.

To recap, shame is the primary emotion. Guilt is added on by humans and is determined by deciding something is right or wrong. Right or wrong are determined by a group of humans with a specific goal or aim. The rules are enacted and are either written or verbal. There is a judge to determine close calls. (For the purposes of this book, I am going to use guilt. But this will imply an underlying shame.)

Guilt is both a powerful tool and a very negative emotion. People with guilt feel bad. People do not like to feel guilt. Humans will do many things to try to rid themselves of guilt. I think a lot of addictions—either with chemicals or behaviors—stem from attempts to cover up the bad feelings that accompany guilt.

One of the worst things about guilt is that it can be permanent. The action or thought that created guilt is in the past, but humans have good memories. There is nothing to make guilt go away once it is created. Our memories keep it alive.

Let's return to my interaction with Maryanne, my patient. Using the definitions we have established, how could I lessen my guilt?

Look at this situation in more detail. Let's use our understanding of right and wrong. Did I do something wrong? To answer that, we need to go back to the definition of right and wrong. We need to look at her group and its rules, goals, and judge. This is not as easy as it sounds.

What group am I in? I am a physician. I have been trained to be accurate. I have been given tools to improve my accuracy. But I am also a human. Humans are known to commit errors.

Next, what are the written and unwritten rules? Doctors are responsible for their patients and the outcome of their interactions. We have rules that are made to ensure doctors do the appropriate amount of investigation to avoid errors. We have a whole malpractice system that has a series of rules and laws to govern the process.

What is the goal? The goal is for a doctor to use all the skills necessary to make an accurate diagnosis and advise the patient of the best course to take.

And who will be the judge? The patient can be a judge here. The medical community and legal community have a system in place to judge cases. These judges—and sometimes juries—are given the power to make decisions on cases that are not clear-cut. I am a judge also. Sometimes the individual is the harshest judge.

All this background discussion leads us to a critical question. *How do I have less guilt?*

Guilt is meant to be a punishment for doing something wrong within a given society that has a set of rules, a goal, and a judge to arbitrate. In understanding your guilt, you first must decide what group you belong to. Once you determine that, you will know the set of rules you must follow.

I had to realize that the groups I belong to all have the concept that no one is perfect. Every human has made mistakes. This is so well recognized that it has reached the status of a proverb in our society: *To err is human.* No one likes to be imperfect. We all want to be right all the time. I had to accept that, to be included in the group of humans, error has to be a part of the equation.

I had to see that I followed "the rules" when it came to evaluating a patient for chest pain. I spoke to the patient. I knew her history of indigestion. I examined the patient. I did the appropriate tests. I communicated my thinking process with Maryanne and decided that this was indigestion, not a heart attack.

Maryanne did not sue me. No official judge was involved in this case. But she and I are clearly judges in this case. By continuing to come to my office and follow my advice, she clearly did not judge me harshly. I had to learn that I was not going to be perfect but that I would be committed to trying to make every decision as accurate as possible. I also talked to my colleagues. I was seeking their advice on whether I had done something wrong. I wanted to learn if there was some other clue or test that I could have done, given the circumstances of Maryanne's case. My colleagues thought I had done all the appropriate tests. They understood my guilt because they, too, had made mistakes in the past.

As an emotion, guilt is meant to punish—but also to change behavior. People feel guilty about what they did, even though it took place in the past and cannot be undone. Their memory keeps the guilt alive. In fact, humans have incredible memory. We can remember things that happened when we were five years old, even when we are ninety-five. We have amazing technology to help us remember. We have videos, photos, writings, computer clouds, and others' memories to remind us what happened in the past. This has both positive and negative implications. We can remember good occurrences, but we can also remember bad things.

Guilt can't change what happened.

It can only change what will happen in the future. In my case, my guilt changed how I handled patients who came to my office with chest pain. My guilt had the effect of changing my behavior in the future. Guilt had done its job. Today, when I see a patient with chest pain, I know that the information I get in the office could lead to a wrong conclusion. I spend extra time with my history and physical. I might do a second EKG; my threshold for sending someone to the hospital is lower. I spend more time talking to the patient about what might happen if all the evidence is wrong and it isn't indigestion but really is a heart attack. I am a better doctor because of this. Beating myself up about Maryanne's heart attack doesn't make her heart get better. It did make me change my behavior, and it made me a more thorough doctor that I have continued to be throughout my career. Guilt did its job and changed my behavior.

If the purpose of guilt is to change behavior in the future, then you are successful if you do not commit the guilt-causing action again. Acknowledging that accomplishment can reduce your feeling of guilt. If you do engage in the offending behavior again, you should feel guilty again. You are doing something wrong, and you are not changing your behavior. This can describe addiction or any negative behavior that is repeated despite negative consequences. This is a topic for my upcoming book, *New Outcomes*. You can refer to the chapter where I talk about change.

The last piece of advice I have for you to reduce or eliminate your guilt is about forgiveness. Human societies use shame and guilt to punish and shape behavior. But they also use forgiveness to recognize when someone has changed and complied with the rules and judge's decision. In all societies, there is a mechanism by which a member can ask and obtain forgiveness. If you did something wrong, you might have to pay a fine or spend time in jail, but when your punishment is over, you are allowed back into society. Most religions have a way for people to ask and receive forgiveness as long as they are willing to commit to changing the offending act. Christianity has Jesus to help alleviate believers' guilt. Buddhism has Karma. Catholicism has confession. But I have been particularly struck by Desmond Tutu and his daughter Mpho, and their prescription for forgiveness.

I would suggest you read *The Book of Forgiving*, by Desmond Tutu and his daughter, Mpho Tutu. It is a book every human should read. The Tutus suggest that humans are all connected, like a fabric, and when someone does something wrong, it creates a tear in the fabric of society. For them, forgiveness is the mending of that tear. The book suggests a four-part process toward forgiveness.

| First, tell your story. |

There is a great psychic cost to keeping a secret. Not only does it take a lot of energy, but the secret erects a barrier between you and the person you are keeping the secret from. That, in turn, makes the guilt fester inside. Of course, the person or group you tell needs to be trustworthy and empathetic. I told my colleagues about my error.

Second, name the hurt.

This validates that something happened and that an element of it was bad. No more hiding it under a rug or in the closet of your mind. I admitted that my mistake led to Maryanne's life changing.

Third, ask for forgiveness.

It is not necessary to receive forgiveness, but it is necessary to ask for it. The asking is the important part. After you have told your story and validated that something bad happened, asking for forgiveness is the crucial next step. This will help you make the changes to make sure the same error is not made again. Getting forgiveness makes you feel better. It lessens the blow. But it is not completely necessary. Your enemy may never forgive you, but, by asking, you have made a commitment to change. In my case, I did not know this part while Maryanne was alive. I asked her forgiveness in my prayers. And on reflection, I realize her coming to me after her heart attack was her way of forgiving me.

Fourth, renew or release the relationship.

This means after you have told your story, named the hurt, and asked for forgiveness, you form a new relationship with the person or group you have wronged. This fourth step is not an easy process. It takes effort. It takes patience. It takes bravery. But the reward of reducing your guilt is worth it. It is how we mend the tear in the fabric of our human society. According to the Tutus, when you go through this process, your existing relationship is changed. Sometimes a new, stronger bond is formed between you and the hurt party because you are operating on a more honest field. Honesty allows people to trust you more. Lying erodes trust. By being honest, you allow yourself and the other person to become more intimate. Your relationship can be renewed and can become even stronger because you were able to find a new level of commitment by being honest and asking forgiveness. Most people want the truth. It may be difficult in the short run, but someone who is willing to be honest—even if it means losing the relationship—will make better relationships in the future.

But this honesty can also mean the end of the existing relationship. The other party may be so hurt or angry that they cannot maintain the relationship. They may never speak to you again. That is the risk you have to take. The Tutus recognize this and tell you sometimes you have to release the current relationship.

I see this play out in marriages where there has been infidelity. When the truth is exposed, two outcomes are possible. Some marriages are actually strengthened. The couple gets counseling, they rediscover why they had gotten married in the first place, they see the infidelity as a symptom of a deteriorating relationship, and they vow to build back their love for each other. They have recommitted to each other and are more honest with each other.

But there are other relationships where there is no more interaction. The tear in the fabric cannot be repaired. Then each person must move on. Leave that relationship in the past, and move on to a new relationship with another human. When you ask for forgiveness, you may not get it, even if you have changed. You have to accept that you cannot change the past. You can only change the future. I see this in patients with addiction. They have gotten sober, but their loved one cannot get over the hurt they felt from the history of lies and abuse. You have to let go, or it becomes a weight that drags on your energy and your self esteem. Find new relationships, but vow never to commit that error again.

This process of forgiveness also means forgiving yourself. You can use the four-step process on yourself. You will need to establish a new way of looking at yourself. You will become someone willing to face your past, your wrongs, and your decisions. You will become someone who accepts that this happened in the past and, because of your strength, never happened again.

I had a patient, a young girl, who witnessed her mother being hit by her father. She tried to stop her dad but was unsuccessful. She felt guilty that she did not do enough to help her mom. We reviewed the scenario. She was willing to tell me the story and name the hurt. She asked her current self for forgiveness. She reframed the story now that she was older. I helped her realize she risked her life to help her mom. She did what heroes do. She was afraid but overcame her fear to help her mom. In the room, my patient had tears well up in her eyes. With her own forgiveness and reframing the scenario, she told me she felt lighter. A weight had been taken off of her. Sometimes the hardest person to ask for and get forgiveness from is yourself.

Desmond Tutu and his daughter write, "There are two simple truths. There is nothing that cannot be forgiven, and there is no one undeserving of forgiveness." I have learned that lesson myself.

It is not my intention to eliminate guilt. Society needs guilt to shape behavior. When a person has no guilt, we label them a sociopath. Society does not want individuals killing others with no sense of guilt. It is dangerous. Guilt is a tool that shapes what people do in the future. What I am trying to accomplish is to help you not make guilt so burdensome that it sucks the energy and self-esteem from your life.

Guilt is meant to change your behavior in the future. If you feel bad about what you did, recognize the part of your behavior that violated the rules of your group, and change your behavior in the future so that you never repeat the offending action. You deserve to feel positive about yourself and your accomplishments. Hold your head high. Recognize your worth and your right to your position in society.

There are other specific treatments that will help people with excessive guilt.

Cognitive behavioral therapy is one. Psychologists use this technique in weekly sessions. It can be very effective. The person uses their cognitive skills to change the predominant thinking to a more helpful thought process. This process can take time to be effective.

Hypnosis and Neurolinguistic Programming can also help reframe the past and establish a basis for improved self-esteem. I did this with my patient. By reframing the scene with her father and mother, she was able to release her guilt and felt lighter.

For some patients, medications can be useful. If your mood is so bad that you cannot function, then changing the chemistry of your brain may be necessary to get you to a level that you are functional and can take advantage of the other modalities.

Now that you have read this chapter and understand guilt, let me know if you can think up any techniques to reduce the effects of guilt. Give me your suggestions on my website, TheLessStressDoc.com.

LET'S RECAP

Definition of Guilt

Guilt is what occurs when the negative emotion from the brain known as shame is combined with the mind's ability to label actions and ideas as right or wrong.

Human Skill: Determining right and wrong
Side Effect: Shame
Tools:

- Defining right and wrong requires you to define a group, a set of rules, a goal, and a judge.

- Guilt is designed to change your behavior in the future.

- To better understand when you are feeling guilty, you should identify the group you are in, acknowledge the rules, and find a judge.

- Recognize that what you have done in the past cannot be changed but that your behavior in the future can be changed. Give yourself credit for not repeating the offense.

- Seek forgiveness. Tell your story, name the hurt, ask for forgiveness, and renew or release your relationship.

- Use this same process to forgive yourself.

- Remember that the goal is not to get rid of guilt. Guilt is necessary for society to function. The goal is to reduce guilt and change your future behavior.

- Cognitive behavioral therapy, hypnosis with Neurolinguistic Programming, and medications are other ways to help reduce excessive guilt.

This chapter is designed to guide you toward less guilt. You will learn to forgive yourself. You will establish a new baseline for your current relationships and perhaps start new ones. You will be able to hold your head high, knowing you have learned from your past and changed your behavior. And, of course, you will spend more time in your Happy Place, with happiness, contentment, and the anticipation of good things to come.

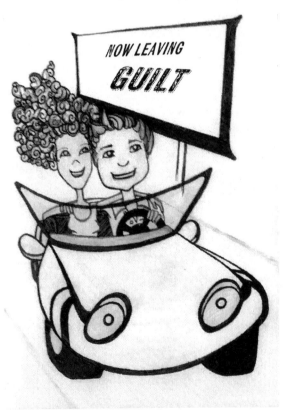

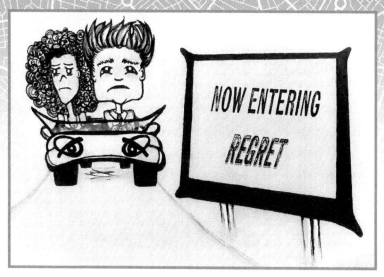

CHAPTER FOUR:

Regret

Are Regrets Over Past Decisions Keeping You From Moving Forward?

In this chapter I will define regret. I will tell you a personal story about my regret. I will show you how regret is different from guilt but also how it is similar. I will show you the three components of choice. I will introduce you to Directed Awareness. I will define good and bad as a concept. Then I will show you that regret is designed to change your future behavior. Identify the process you went through to make your decision. Separate the process from the result. Understand that choices are made without all the information you would like to have. Don't go back up the decision tree. Who else is deciding on the decision besides you? I will also touch on therapy, medication, and NLP.

Definition of Regret: Regret is a secondary negative emotion built on the primary emotions of sadness and/or anger that comes from making a bad choice/decision in the past.

I'm going to use me again. I wish I didn't have any personal stories that would illustrate my points, but I guess I really am just a human.

After years of marriage, I got divorced. I don't regret that. I have had time to reflect on that, and I've realized that my ex-wife and I had changed over the years; we no longer matched up.

My regret had to do with my kids. During the divorce, I wanted it to be kid-centric. Whatever was good for the kids was worth doing. Whatever wasn't good for the kids wasn't worth doing. As an example, my lawyer advised me to have the family house sold, so that my ex-wife could not use the house as a weapon. This would have meant my kids would have to move to a new house. I refused. I wanted them to have the least amount of disruption. My decision cost me in some ways, but it was worth it for the kids.

What I regretted was how I left. I had a plan. I would tell my ex-wife I wanted a divorce. I decided I would get an apartment and allow her to stay in the house with the children. But I wanted the children to have a month to get used to the idea of my leaving. I envisioned a family meeting where I told them that, in a month I would be moving out to a nearby apartment. My ex-wife could not abide by that. We couldn't agree on a plan together, so we hired a referee and agreed to abide by his decision. The referee was a psychologist who was familiar to us. We went to see him, and, after hearing our story, he concluded that my wife could not tolerate me being in the house knowing I was going to be divorcing her. He decided that, for her sake—and by extension, my kids' sake—that I should leave immediately.

We had the family meeting. I told the kids that I would be divorcing Mom. I would be living in a nearby apartment. And, to be true to my agreement with my ex-wife, the next day, I left. I did not think it was a good decision at the time, and I still don't. It is a regret I have to live with. I was angry at the choice that I had made. I was also feeling sad for my kids and how this would color their image of me as a father. I wish I could do it over again—because I would do it differently—but that is the problem with the past. It is done and can't be changed.

I don't know how many of you are parents who have been through a divorce, but even if that is not your regret, I'm sure you have some regrets in your life. The question that is before us is, *How can we get rid of—or, at least, reduce—the regret?*

Regret is different from guilt. Guilt is based on breaking the rules, either stated or unstated. Guilt is doing something wrong or committing an error. It has a base of shame and a topping of wrong. Regret is not connected to shame. I didn't break any rules. In fact, I was doing what a psychologist thought would be the best for the kids. I felt it was the wrong choice and that there was a better choice to make.

I don't understand. Can you go into more detail about what makes regret different than guilt?

Of course. Guilt and regret are similar in that they are emotions based on something that happened in the past. The past could be minutes or years, but the important part is that the action has already occurred when we decide how to feel about it. Both guilt and regret make you feel bad; in both cases, you want to limit the bad feeling. The difference is that guilt is based on doing something wrong. Regret is based on making a bad choice. The choice doesn't have to be wrong or illegal, but it leads to an outcome that was not as good as it could have been. If you had made a different choice, things might have turned out better.

Regret happens as you look back on a situation and then make a value judgment of whether you made the optimum choice. Regret can be experienced only by humans because only humans have the ability to choose and then assign the concept of good or bad. My daughter's dog, Huxley, might not eat the food she gave him because it doesn't taste good, but he doesn't think of it as bad. He just doesn't eat it.

Choice seems to be the important part of regret. Can you define it better?

You're catching on. A concept should be defined in a concrete, usable way. Good for you.

The ability to choose is a game changer. It has literally changed the environment of the Earth. In the past, there was geology. Then biology came along. There were billions of years for these two entities to merge into balance. Then humans added choice to the environment. Now humans can choose to cut down the rainforest for wood to build a house. No, on second thought, humans won't cut down the forest. We will build our houses out of stone. In a future book, I plan to go into the philosophy behind Stratastheres in greater detail. For now, let me answer your question about how we define choice.

As you guessed, choice is not as easy as it sounds. Choice requires three things.

1. Directed awareness

2. Alternatives

3. Good and bad

Directed awareness is a term I use now. Not only have I found "conscious," "subconscious," and "unconscious" to be terms too hard to define, but I don't think they have an anatomical basis. The term "directed awareness" allows me to make more sense of what goes into choice for humans.

In my world, directed awareness is the human ability to focus on a particular brain tract or memory. If I ask you what two plus two equals, your directed awareness points you to another part of your brain/memory, and you answer "four." It was immediate, and you did not need any clues. You have direct access to this information. I'm assuming that there is an anatomical structure in the brain that allows humans to have directed awareness. It is probably in the frontal lobe. This same structure allows for self-awareness.

Other animals do not have this skill, or, if they do, it is limited when compared to humans'. I believe it is an anatomical structure because I have seen patients who have had a stroke; they no longer have self-awareness. They can't tell their left arm from their right arm. (Really.) I also think directed awareness develops over time. Infants do not have directed awareness. I believe this explains why we can't remember much of what happened before age five—the structure responsible for directed awareness hasn't fully developed yet. We can make memories, but we can't retrieve them.

Directed awareness is vitally important for humans. You can direct your brain and mind to focus on a particular memory or concept or to focus on a particular body part or object in your environment. When you are making a decision, you can use directed awareness to bring up the pros and cons of a given choice. You can use your access to memory to bring forward information that will help you in making a decision. Humans have a huge capacity for memory; it is enhanced by using concepts and technology. Concepts allow a word like "door" to stand for a whole array of objects that act like a door. It is a kind of shorthand. Technology refers to the tools you use—writing implements, photographs, books, computers. You can bring a lot of information to the table to aid in your choice.

Factors other than directed awareness also enter into your process for choosing. Directed awareness is great, but it is limited. Some memories and concepts are connected to directed awareness, but you need a hint to find them. This is what occurs when you are trying to remember the name of the fellow you just met. You made the memory but can't retrieve it. Your spouse says it's "Bob," but that isn't right. You overhear the person next to you talking about Jimmy Kimmel. *That's it. His name is Jim.* You know that is the right answer. You just needed a hint to find it. Google has become the great source for hints. When you are having a dinner discussion about movies with a particular star, Google will remind you of all the movies that star acted in. Many were already in your memory, but you needed the Google hint to find them.

There are other parts of your brain to which you have no direct access. Your brain is monitoring your thyroid level, your growth-hormone level, the speed of your heart rate, and the carbon dioxide in your bloodstream. But you have no access to this information. It is not connected to your directed awareness. When someone tells you we only use 10 percent of our brain, I believe that is incorrect. We use all of our brain all of the time. But we might have direct awareness of only 10 percent of our brain. Since there are parts of your brain that are working but to which you have no direct access, there can be influences on your decisions that you are not aware of.

There was a study done by William and Bargh. In it, the researcher rode up the elevator with his research subject to an interview room. The subject was unaware that the fellow rider in the elevator was the study coordinator. He assumed he was just a fellow traveler in the elevator. The study coordinator gave the research subject either a cold soda or a hot cup of coffee. When the subject got off the elevator, he or she went to a room where they were instructed to interview someone and rate how "warm" the personality traits were. It turned out that subjects given a cold beverage were less likely to describe the person as "warm." Subjects given a hot beverage were more likely to find the person "warm." What?! The study coordinators were shocked by this finding and didn't believe it was real. They repeated the study multiple times and in multiple ways, and it kept showing the same results.

In my interpretation, the subjects were influenced by something outside their direct awareness. This is also the basis for subliminal messaging. There is a reason that women buy beauty products from beautiful women and men buy sports cars that advertise with a sexy woman draped over the hood. When humans make a choice, they receive influences from both their directed awareness and the rest of the brain.

Directed awareness is the first requirement for there to be choice. The second requirement is alternatives. If there is no alternative, there is no choice. If the path goes only one way, you can go only one way. If there is a fork in the path, then you can choose to go down the one less traveled. (What would Robert Frost have written if there had been no fork and, thus, no roads to choose between?)

Generally, humans face lots of alternatives. How many kinds of beer or hot sauce can there be? In fact, we probably have too many choices. When Alvin Toffler wrote *Future Shock* in 1970, he described what happens when there are too many alternatives. That was more than fifty years ago. We have even more choices today—and having too many choices is a stressor. It takes energy to make a choice. It takes time and brain energy. Thinking isn't free. When I was on call in the past, I would get a hundred phone calls in two days. Each phone call necessitated a choice. After about seventy-five phone calls, I was starting to feel overwhelmed. The last ten phone calls were a struggle. My life is easier now. A weekend on call might mean twenty phone calls. I can handle that.

That brings us to the third requirement for choice to exist: the concept of good and bad. The human-created idea of good and bad differs from that of right and wrong. Right and wrong are about rules and judges. Good and bad are not as concrete.

I looked up "good," and there were fifty-nine separate definitions. ("Bad" had only forty-eight—I'm not sure if there is significance to that distinction.) In the framework of choice, *good* somehow leads to a better outcome, while *bad* is the opposite. Good/bad does have similarity to right/wrong in that they are both defined within a cultural context. What is good in one culture or group might lead to a bad outcome in another setting. Good/bad can change quickly. Something that is good one day can be bad the next, and vice versa.

Good and bad also need a goal, much like right and wrong—perhaps even more so since *outcome* is really part of the definition of good and bad. A defined goal is important in distinguishing good from bad. Since good and bad are related to outcome, there is also a difference between short-term goals and long-term goals. Going to college can be bad in the short run. It is time consuming and expensive. But in the long term, it is good because it enables you to earn more money and to accomplish more, which gives you better self-esteem. (There is more about this in the chapter on self-esteem.)

All organisms are set up to make short-term decisions. Most don't have a future, so a long-term decision is not a possibility. Humans, however, have a future. That means long-term goals exist for humans. Even though that is true, we are still organisms with a default position focused on short-term goals. You need to get to work today, so you drive your car. However, given that greenhouse gases are causing global warning, you should really ride your bike to work. That would be the good long-term choice.

Good can also change in retrospect. A father is concerned that his 18-year-old son broke his leg. That is bad. But the next day, a recruiter for the Army comes to town to recruit 18-year-olds to go to war. This man's son is passed over because he has a broken leg. That is good.

All this takes us back to our original stressor, which is regret. Regret, like guilt, is based on something in the past. However, your negative feelings about it are occurring in the present—and those negative feelings will continue to plague you as long as you have memory about the decision you made or as long as technology keeps allowing you to recall what happened. Regret can go on indefinitely. This is not very encouraging.

Although regret is different from guilt, the two often go hand in hand—which is why they can be confused. If I decide to rob a bank, I am doing something against the rules and should feel guilty. But I am also making a bad decision. I am a smart guy and could probably figure out how to rob a bank and not get caught immediately. In the short term, my desire to have more money and the things that come with that wealth would be satisfied. In the long term, however, I might get caught and go to jail. I would lose the money and even more. I will regret my decision to rob the bank instead of going to work and earning money the legal way.

Regret is about decisions, and decisions tend to be based on previous decisions. To see your previous choices, you can trace back along the branches of the tree that contains all your decisions prior to this regrettable one. In my story, I can focus on the decision to leave the house the day after telling my kids that their parents were getting a divorce. I can back up and regret agreeing to a referee. I could go back to the decision to leave my wife. I could go back even further and ask why I married her in the first place. I can go back as far as I like to find a choice that could have altered the outcome.

Humans have that ability to track back into their past decisions and use them to their detriment all the time.

If that is regret, how can I have less of it?

Now that we have fleshed out the three components of choice, let's refresh the definition of regret. **Regret is a secondary negative emotion built on the primary emotions of sadness**

and/or anger that comes from making a bad choice/decision in the past.

As with guilt, I don't want you to get rid of regret. By providing a valuable negative reinforcement, it allows humans to learn from their past. You should feel regret if you make a bad decision. Regret helps influence what you do in the future. It comes from a decision that was bad (although not necessarily wrong).

I'll give you a different personal example. I was trying to decide on a computer system for my office. I did research and talked to the people working for me. I examined my budget. I looked into the future to consider the impact my decision would have on me and the office. One factor in my decision was my current office manager, who was very familiar with computer Brand A. She had used this computer in her previous job, and it worked well. My other staff members had no experience with Brand A, but they were willing to learn from someone who did. This particular computer fit with my budget and met the needs of my office.

My only concern was what would happen if I invested in that type of computer and my office manager left. The rest of my staff would be trying to learn to use this computer system without a teacher. I raised this concern with my office manager. She told me she had no plans to leave. She was happy in this job and had even turned down jobs that paid her $10 more per hour. With that reassurance, I bought the computer Brand A. However, the computer had not been delivered yet when my office manager came to me, upset, to say she had been given an unsolicited offer from another office. She would earn $20 more an hour than I paid her. She had decided to take the new job.

My purchase of computer Brand A was starting to look like a bad decision.

Who decides if this is a bad decision? I have a say, but my staff also gets to weigh in, and they felt it was a bad decision. They were put in the position of having to learn a new computer system with no in-house teacher. It made for a difficult transition. Their lives had been negatively impacted. I, on the other hand, had a different opinion. The outcome was not what I wanted, but, when I reviewed my decision-making process given the information I had at the time, I felt it had been a good decision. The decision became bad only when the circumstances changed.

This is an important distinction. When trying to mitigate regret, you need to remember that you made your decision based on the available information *at the time*. Looking into the future to try to avoid negative outcomes is not an exact science. Maybe you don't have sufficient experience or haven't learned enough from the past experiences you do have. None of us are that great at predicting the future.

To lessen your feeling of regret, you should think about the information you had at the time, think about your past experiences, and consider—given those two things—whether you made the most logical decision. If you had it to do over again, knowing what you did then, would you make the same decision? If so, you did not make a bad decision. You simply made a decision that didn't turn out as you expected, because you were working with shifting information and a spotty ability to predict the future.

I referred to the coronavirus earlier. There was clearly not enough information available at the onset of the pandemic. Past experience was helpful, but the world's connectivity had changed since the previous pandemic. Who would have predicted that a small percentage of sick people in China would force the entire world into quarantine? Public health leaders should not regret any decisions they made that were attuned to information available at the time. That is not to say public health officials (and the rest of us) can't learn. If there was a bad outcome, you learn from that. You can revise the decision-making process you use, or you can include other sources of information the next time you decide.

Back to me and the computer purchase. At the time I bought the computer, my office manager showed significant loyalty. If I had known she was going to leave, I would have made a different decision. Her continuing presence in the office was critical to my computer choice. If she had stayed, my decision would have had a good outcome, and my staff would have agreed with it. Because I realize all this, I have less regret about my decision. Nonetheless, I learned from it. The next time a decision came up about buying an upgraded computer system, I made my office manager sign in blood that she would not leave. OK, I didn't really make her sign in blood, but I did not put myself in the position where I needed to rely exclusively on my new office manager's computer experience. Furthermore, I gave greater weight to my other employees' input.

Here's how you mitigate regret. You look at the process you used en route to your decision. If it was good, you should feel less regret. If it didn't have a good outcome, you can learn, change your decision-making process, or collect more information to try to get a better outcome next time. The other thing you can do is avoid going back up that tree of decisions. It is a trap that only leads to more regret. That's because you can always find a branch on that tree where you should have made a different decision in order to get the outcome you desired. The *past* has already happened. You can't change it.

Like guilt, regret's real power comes from changing your *future* behavior. So, stop wasting your energy on feeling sad, angry, or regretful about past decisions. You also need to revel in your ability to make a choice. Being able to choose is a luxury that no other animal has. You can choose a blue car or a red car, or you can choose a motorcycle, or you can walk. You can read any of a million books or listen to a million songs. I can talk to a person in Iceland or Thailand. I can travel to those places and actually meet face-to-face with my Icelandic or Thai friend with whom I have been Skyping. As my next-door neighbor reminds me, "Gary, how great is this day!"

Don't get caught up in feeling bad about one decision. Just learn from the past, and change your behavior as you move into the future. This has been said by so many great people, including people who posted more failures than successes. They recognized that the process they were going through was good, regardless of the outcomes. They saw the decisions they made as a necessary step toward success. Learn and move on. There is the wonder of the world out there to enjoy.

I will repeat that there are other therapies that are out there for your benefit. If you want other ways to reduce your regret, you can see a therapist who uses cognitive behavioral therapy.

Hypnosis and NLP can be excellent tools to disencumber emotions from your memories. Reframing the memory to exclude the negative emotion can be very helpful.

If you still find it hard to move out of the cycle of regret, there are also medications that can be effective under a doctor's supervision. That would need to be brought up with your own personal physician.

Now that you have read this chapter and understand regret, let me know if you can think up any techniques for having less regret. Give me your suggestions on my website, TheLessStressDoc.com.

LET'S RECAP

Definition of Regret

Regret is a secondary negative emotion built on the primary emotions of sadness and/or anger that comes from making a bad choice/decision in the past.

Human Skill: Ability to choose, determining good and bad
Side effect: Sadness, anger
Tools:

- Choice is made up of three components. They are directed awareness, alternatives, and the concept of good and bad. You cannot have choice if you do not have these three elements.

- Directed awareness allows purposeful access to the information in our brain.

- We have a lot of alternatives, when you have too many alternatives it is worth paring them down.

- Define good as a better outcome; bad is the opposite.

- Keep in mind that regret is about the past. It could surface within seconds of a choice, or it could appear years later, but it is always about the past. And like guilt, what is in the past can't be changed.

- Regret often goes hand in hand with guilt.

- Don't try to eliminate all regret but limit its impact and use it to change your responses in the future. Don't beat yourself up when you have changed your decision-making process or you have new information that would have changed your behavior.

- To help lessen regret, figure out who gets to weigh in on whether your decision was good or not.

- When you make a decision, remember you are limited by the information you have, the past experience you have, and your inability to predict the future.

- Think about the process and information you used to make a decision. If there was a bad outcome, decide if it was a process problem or an information problem. If it was because information changed or the environment changed, you do not need to regret your decision/choice.

- Avoid going back up the decision tree. If you go back far enough, you can always find a bad decision to make you feel bad.

- Revel in your human ability to choose and the success of humans to have alternatives.

- Therapists and medications are available if the above isn't as successful as you would like.

Now that you understand what causes regret, you can give find ways to lessen the negative effect of regret. There will always be decisions that lead to a bad outcome, but these should be seen as necessary setbacks on the path to your desired goal. Reducing regret will allow you to spend more time in your Happy Place and look forward to the pleasures life can bring.

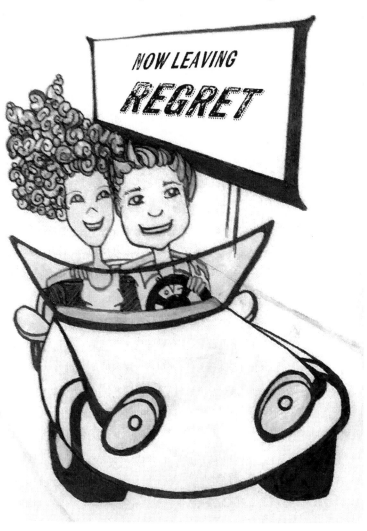

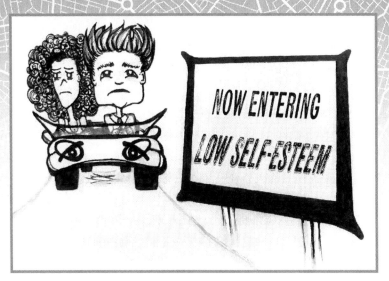

CHAPTER FIVE

Low Self-Esteem

Self-Esteem Isn't Only Self

This chapter will define the three components of self-esteem: self-worth, self-respect, and self-efficacy. I will introduce you to Mandy. I will explain how you process information in your brain/mind. I will introduce a "Perspective Prism." Self-esteem is a core concept. Then I will explore good and bad a little further. I will explain that self-esteem isn't only about self but that the group is also involved in a large way. There is a "Group vs. Me" meter in our head. I will show the scoring scheme for accomplishments and your labeled portrait. To improve self-esteem, you have to be willing to change a core concept. Count your accomplishments and your defining characteristics accurately.

Stop taking your accomplishments and your successes for granted. Make a new tract.

Definition of self-esteem: Self-esteem is an individual's accumulated judgment of their own self-worth, self-respect, and self-efficacy. Self-worth is the answer to the question "Am I a good person or a bad person?" Self-respect is a measure of whether a person is doing things the right way. Self-efficacy is a confidence measurement linked to an individual's ability to accomplish a task in the future.

Mandy is a bright lady who started working with computers when their total memory was 256K. Despite that technological limitation, she had the perseverance and the skill to make brochures for clients. The clients were amazed at her ability to use the available software to craft beautiful, perfectly arranged brochures that could be printed and given to their customers. Mandy was often told how good she was, how smart she was, how irreplaceable she was. But she knew those comments were wrong.

At home after work, Mandy viewed the accolades as a faded, inaccurate treasure map that led to nowhere. She felt that she was pretending to be competent, and she was waiting for the day when everyone else learned she wasn't that good or found someone to replace her. She often thought of suicide to end the charade. She even tried it once. She took a bottle of Tylenol and waited for her liver to fail. She told someone she had taken the whole bottle, but they didn't seem to care. After three days and no evidence of yellow jaundice to indicate liver damage, Mandy realized she'd failed at committing suicide, too. Oh, well, it fit her pattern of inadequacy. Chalk it up to another bit of evidence that she sucked. Clearly, Mandy had low self-esteem.

Why is self-esteem so important?

Your self-esteem plays a role in how you see things, how you feel, and how you act. It is literally involved in how you process every piece of information you are exposed to. It is a powerful concept that can lead to happiness and success or to sadness, guilt, regret, and failure. We all have some sense of self-esteem, and it is constantly being challenged by our environment and our decisions. Self-esteem is an inner, core sphere of your "Perspective Prism." Every bit of information that hits your sensory awareness first goes through your Perspective Prism, where self-esteem fills the center.

Wait, what is a "Perspective Prism"?

This is a concept I have been using on myself and with my patients. The Perspective Prism is an explanation for why two people can see the same scene and come away with totally different perceptions. Let me go into some more detail.

Perspective Prism

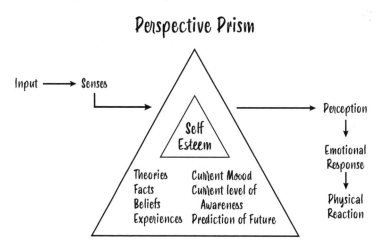

The above graph is a shorthand way to see how our brains and minds process information and lead to reactions. This is the basis for most thinking and most behavior.

Input can be anything from the external environment. A noise, a smell, a picture, a scene. It can also be from our internal environment. A skipped heartbeat, chest pain, a muscle twitch, a headache. These inputs are constantly bombarding our system. Most of the information is ignored or processed by the unaware part of our brain. Very little is actually brought to the directed-awareness portion. The temperature of the room is not part of my awareness until it becomes too hot or too cold.

The input is processed by our Perspective Prism. Inside each of our Perspective Prisms are a number of entities. There is our self-esteem, facts we believe, our theories, our past experiences, our predictions of future events, things we believe but can't prove, our emotional state, our state of awareness.

This prism is layered. In the central core are determinations of self-esteem, believing in a higher power, and other central tenets. There are outer spheres that are dependent on the core. The outer sphere is based on the inner sphere. I pray because I believe in God. If I believe in God, then praying to God makes sense. If I don't believe in God, then praying to God makes no sense.

Anything in our prism can be changed. Some are easier to change than others. I might think holes in my jeans are a sign I am poor. Then, again, I might think holes in my jeans are a sign I am fashion-conscious and have a lot of money. But other ideas are more difficult to change. Self-esteem is a central, core concept and is difficult (but possible) to change. Believing in a higher power or not is a difficult one to change. The Earth is round, the Earth rotates around the sun, Newton was wrong,

Einstein was right, Darwin and God can coexist. All the facts and theories we hold in our prism can be changed.

Each one of us has a prism, and each one is different. Now, when input comes from the external or internal environment, it is filtered through the Perspective Prism. What comes out on the other side is our perception. Our perception is what we use to decide our reaction to any given input. Here is an example: I am in the exam room with a patient, and my nurse walks in with a large syringe with a long, thick needle. In my patient's prism is the theory that *That needle is for me.* I see the exact same thing, but I know the needle is for the patient in the next room. We see the same thing, but our prisms are different, and so our perception is different.

Our perceptions then drive our reactions. Our perceptions set off emotional responses or a thinking process. The perception will change, depending on the Perspective Prism. In this example, my patient's perception is that the needle is meant for her, and she reacts with fear. My perception is that the nurse is in the wrong room, and she is causing distress with the patient in this room. My reaction is annoyance bordering on anger. Same input, different perceptions, and different emotional responses.

The last step is reacting. Based on the input, Perspective Prism, perception, and emotional response, I now have to react. It could be a physical reaction or a mental reaction. In this example, my patient is afraid, and she retreats to the back of the room, away from the needle. I have a different reaction. I am not afraid. I calmly (hopefully) tell the nurse she is in the wrong room.

This pattern can be used to describe any behavior you see. The biggest variable is the Perspective Prism. This is where there is a lot of information stored from the past and the expected future. If I just got of jail and I hear a siren, I'm thinking the police are coming to arrest me again. My perception is different if I am being robbed at knifepoint and hear a siren. I think the police are on their way to help me.

The Perspective Prism is what we use to understand ourselves and others. The more I know about my own prism, the more I can understand my behavior. In the same way, the more I know about your prism, the more I can understand why you react the way you do. Self-exploration and empathy really boil down to the same thing—what is in a person's perspective prism.

Bringing this discussion back to self-esteem, your Perspective Prism was being formed from your infancy. Each input was laying the foundation for what you think of yourself, your self-worth, your self-respect, and your self-efficacy. As the foundation was being laid down, it was also being used as a filter to determine the significance of new information. This is why it is self-fulfilling. If you start thinking of yourself in bad terms, you will filter the input, and your perception will lean toward the bad, and vice versa.

If self-esteem is so important, why don't I think about it very much?

Since it is a core sphere and it doesn't change much, self-esteem is in the background. It is like the air. It is everywhere and essential, but you never notice it until it isn't there. In addition, I feel it was shaped before your directed awareness was fully developed. Self-esteem starts from the time you first realize that you are separate from your surroundings.

Newborns do not recognize there is a difference between themselves and their environment. Any stranger could hold a three-day-old infant, and the infant will not be able to tell the difference between the stranger and the infant's mother or father. But, as the newborn's brain develops, the baby begins to distinguish between itself, its parents, and others. Try picking up a one-year-old if you are a stranger to that child. The baby's danger response goes off, and you are left with a shattered eardrum from a screaming baby.

This separation of yourself from everyone else is the first skill that must be in place for self-esteem. Newborns don't have this; neither do certain stroke patients. After certain kinds of strokes, patients cannot separate themselves from others. It is a curious situation when I am holding the left hand of a stroke victim who cannot distinguish whether it is my hand or theirs. There is a part of every human brain that is associated with the skill of separating oneself from the environment around us. It develops after birth, and it can be damaged.

Self-esteem also relies on the concept of good and bad. You can't have good self-esteem or bad self-esteem without the concept of good and bad. Put another way, bad self-esteem is the side effect to having the ability to decide something is either good or bad. My dog has a scar on his back. He does not have the concept of good or bad, so he can look at his reflection and see the scar, but he doesn't think it makes him look bad or ugly. He doesn't see his weight gain as a bad thing. He just eats what he can. Nature and his brain will take care of the rest.

Why do we have good and bad?

We talked about good and bad in the chapter on regret, but I want to go further with the discussion. One reason we have good and bad is because we are a communal organism. We have to live within a group, our pack. Our very survival as a species is predicated on the fact that we can work together. We are not very fast, don't have sharp claws, we are not that strong for our size, and we are big but not that big. We survived because we could work together. We could bring the power of 50 against one. But when we work in a group, there has to be a way to coordinate our activities. *Right* and *wrong—good* and *bad*—points us in that direction.

Right and wrong must be a brain function, because other animals have shame. They have a characteristic reaction when doing something they have been taught is wrong. Humans do, too. But we have taken it a step further. A concept of *good* and *bad* comes from our mind skills. It develops only with time and maturation, and it can be lost. Newborns and patients with late-stage Alzheimer's have no concept of good and bad. Babies can throw up all over our new shirt and think nothing of it. Alzheimer's patients wear plaids and stripes together and are not embarrassed.

Good and *bad* are concepts that the group uses to increase the likelihood something will or will not happen. *Good* and *bad* are another way society molds behavior within the group. Early humans lived in bands of fifty or so. It might have been easier for them to define *good* and *bad*, but they also probably had less leeway. Today, we live in bands of millions. It is still necessary to have *good* and *bad* (albeit harder to define them), but there is also more latitude around the concepts. That's because within the millions of people, you can find a subset that thinks what you are doing is *good*, even if the overall group thinks it is *bad*.

Good and *bad* are concepts that help a group of humans survive. It enables them to be more successful in navigating their environment. But the group defines *good* and *bad*, not the individual. This is one of the problems with self-esteem. The individual can affect the group's determination, but the group is the ultimate arbiter of *good* and *bad*. So, self-esteem is not entirely about self. The group has a lot of input.

No matter how many books or therapists tell you to feel good about yourself, no matter how much you rail against *The Man*, it is ultimately the group that has a big say in your self-esteem—like it or not.

To repeat: Self-esteem exists because we can separate ourselves from others, and we have the ability to determine *good* and *bad*. Still, self-esteem is, in large part, shaped by the group we are in.

How does an individual decide if they have good or bad self-esteem?

Once a human has the skill to see himself as a separate entity and can grasp *right/wrong* and *good/bad*, the process begins. Every interaction with the environment starts to lay down the foundation for whether the individual has good or bad self-esteem. I hope you can see the inherent problem here. Your environment, which is dominated by your family, has a lot to say about your self-esteem. *They* are defining *right/wrong, good/bad* when you are too young to do it yourself. If you live in a family that is nurturing and consistent, you will most likely do what family members call *good*. If you live in a family that is not nurturing and consistent, you will most likely do what family members realize is *bad*. As long as you hold your family and close connections as reliable and credible, you will be indoctrinated into their vision of the world. Just as you learn English if you are born in Chester, Maryland, and French if you live in Paris, France, you will learn *good* and *bad* from the influential people around you.

The second problem is your brain, and, hence, your mind is not fully functional when you are young. The perceptions you have as a two-year-old are vastly different than the perceptions of a sixty-year-old. But the sixty-year-old is stuck with the perceptions the two-year-old learned at age two. The determination of self-esteem started at age two, when the brain and mind were easily influenced. Once anatomical tracts/neural pathways are laid down, they are hard to change or rewrite. *I am a good person/I am a bad person* is a tract that is a physical neuron connected to another neuron. These pathways/tracts become so rutted that they feel impossible to change—one, because they were laid at such a young age and, two, because neither individuals nor scientists can get rid of anatomical tracts. The best you can do is make a new tract. There are two other reasons why it feels hard to change the tract: because you rarely examine your self-esteem and because most people don't know or don't think you can change self-esteem once it is established.

As I said earlier, self-esteem is in the core sphere. Every interaction with the environment, every emotion, every perception, every decision is dependent on this core value. Your self-esteem—good or bad—colors every judgment you make. In general, every decision you make is filtered through your self-esteem.

Once self-esteem is established, it becomes a self-fulfilling prophecy. Self-esteem, whether good or bad, affects how every bit of information is processed. When information is presented that is contrary to their belief, people go through a process to rectify the dissonance. They can decide they were wrong and change their mind. But that takes a lot of effort and time. More commonly, people employ methods that enable them to ignore the contrary information. In our initial example, Mandy was an expert at this. There are four ways we do this. I call them the "4 Ds."

The 4 Ds

- **Deny**

- **Deflect**

- **Diminish**

- **Dismiss**

One D is *deny* or *ignore*. If someone says you are a nice person and you have poor self-esteem, you can deny or ignore what they are saying. It doesn't fit your reality, so you simply act as if it didn't happen. Mandy would simply not hear when a co-worker complimented her on a job well done.

The second D is *deflect*. Someone calls you a nice person, and you start talking about a movie you saw last week. The compliment is dissonant with your core belief, so you change the subject to avoid an unpleasant situation. Mandy would talk about computers when she got uncomfortable. If someone was complimenting her on her skills, she would deflect and talk about the computer as a way to change the conversation.

The third D is *diminish*. You can politely thank the person for their compliment, but, in your head, you know they are exaggerating. There were a lot smarter people than her. The person giving her a compliment clearly didn't realize she wasn't that good.

The final D is *dismiss*. Mandy knew the information was inaccurate and assumed the person had an ulterior motive. (My wife says her BS meter goes off). Maybe they want some money or sex—otherwise, why would someone give her a compliment?

The 4 Ds can work in the opposite direction, too. If you have good self-esteem and you are faced with criticism, you use the

4 Ds to counteract the dissonance. You tend to deny, deflect, diminish, or dismiss the critical information that runs contrary to your perceived good self-esteem.

That is how bad and good self-esteem become self-fulfilling. When you have good self-esteem and someone says you are a good person, it fits with the image you carry of yourself, and you agree. If they tell you that you are a bad person, you are likely to employ the 4 Ds. If you have poor self-esteem and the opposite occurs—someone tells you that you are a good person—you turn to the 4 Ds to try to reconcile the conflict. You deny, deflect, diminish, or dismiss. Compliments do not fit. When someone tells you that you are bad, you might dislike the characterization but believe it fits. So, you grumble and see it as further proof of your poor self-image.

It is difficult to process information that runs counter to what you have known since you were two years old and what the most influential people in your life have told you. Yikes. This doesn't sound good for someone who has low self-esteem. But wait. I wouldn't be here talking about self-esteem if I didn't have some answers. I have shown you what self-esteem is and where it comes from. With that information under your belt, I can give you better tools to use to improve your self-esteem, and you can get better results.

What can I do to change my self-esteem?

The first step to changing long-held low self-esteem is to be open to change. Low self-esteem is not something created yesterday or last year. It started when you were two years old or earlier. The tracts have been in place for a long time. The ruts are deep. They are anatomical. Neither you nor the medical profession can get rid of the old tracts. You have been looking through your own self-esteem lens for most of your entire life. Changing that view is a big deal.

Among other things, change is scary, especially when you are talking about a core value. As you have read, when you change an inner, core value, you affect literally everything else in your environment—your past, your future, your emotions, your facts, your beliefs, and so on. This can be daunting. In working with one of my first patients with poor self-esteem, I felt proud of myself. I had expertly dissected her self-esteem problem. I showed her the path to better self-esteem, and I was waiting for a gush of appreciation from her. When I stopped talking long enough to look at her, I was taken aback. In front of me was not an ecstatic woman with a newfound love for herself. In front of me was a lady who looked like she had just been punched in the stomach. What the heck happened? She looked at me and said, "If I have been wrong about myself all these years, what else have I been wrong about?"

I had to think about that for a while. Though you're changing only one fact in your brain, a re-evaluation of your self-esteem changes everything else. That can be disorienting. But, believe me, it is worth it. Learning how to have good self-esteem pays you dividends for the rest of your life. It also benefits your children and the other people around you. It is a glorious day when you can say with conviction, "I really think a lot of me."

Are you willing to try to learn a new way to look at yourself?

From our earlier discussion, you learned that the tracts were set down when you were young. You and I can't change that. But you can lay down new tracts. And you can interact with your new tracts till your response becomes automatic. This is like learning how to be optimistic or learning how to live without cigarettes. It is possible. It's not easy, but it's easier when you know what you are trying to accomplish.

The good news is that you are amazingly smart compared to the rest of the animal kingdom. You can learn something so quickly that you leave all other animals in your dust. You are a supercharged, super-fast sports car. The next animal has a rubber-band wind-up engine in comparison. So, smile and appreciate your skill of learning fast. And now use it. Learn something new. Learn what self-esteem is, learn what you have to do to change it, and practice your new tract of good self-esteem until it is just as deeply dug and well established as your old tract was. This is the first step. Nothing will change if you don't do this. I will talk about this more in Chapter Eight. I can spend all afternoon with you and teach you a lot of interesting things, but nothing will change until you are open to change and put in the work to make a new tract.

Next you must understand that self-esteem is not just about the self. Whatever group you are in also has a say in your self-esteem. The group could be your family, your state, your country, your community club, your baseball team, your reading group, your AA meeting. Whatever group it may be, it has its own *right/wrong* and *good/bad* that influences your evaluation of what is good and bad in you. You might think it is a good idea to ban guns, but if you are in the NRA, you will be viewed as bad, and others in the group will try to kick you out. Every book I read on self-esteem says that you shouldn't worry what other people think, that you should just love yourself as yourself. This sounds nice, but it is both impossible and dangerous. As a group, we want people to follow along. We allow for individuality but only within a small bandwidth. Too much variance, and you are given a clear mandate to change or be shunned.

How do you build up your self-esteem if it isn't all in your control?
Glad you asked.

First, I want to explain the meter we all have inside of us. It is the "Me vs. Group" credibility meter. The meter fluctuates between me having credibility and the group having credibility. On one end is a narcissist or psychopath who takes into consideration only their own needs. The group has no bearing on what they do or think. Next are the geniuses and mavericks. They point the needle toward themselves but not to the exclusion of others. They are thinking outside the normal boundaries of their group. Each group needs a certain number of these individuals because they bring with them a way to change the group. Einstein told scientists that what they had based all their theories and all their research on for 300 years was wrong. Figures like Darwin, Jesus, Mahatma Gandhi, and Martin Luther King, Jr., were all willing to push the needle toward what they believed was good/right. But they stayed within the group and brought the group along. The result was that they changed the group's definition of right/good. This takes a lot more courage, conviction, and perseverance than most of us have.

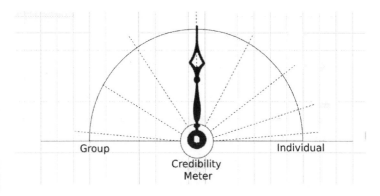

Group   Individual

Credibility
Meter

The meter also has a middle group and endpoint group. The middle group is by far the biggest segment. The people in this group have individual needs and wants but are usually squashing them down because the group's power is enough to keep them from becoming independent thinkers. The endpoint segment is made up of people with low credibility. For them, what the group thinks is what they think. Their opinion doesn't matter at all. Good and bad or right and wrong are defined by the group, with no input from these people. The endpoint group members are constantly checking in with the people around them, seeking approval.

It is not my goal to make you a narcissist or a genius/maverick. I just want you to slide over to the middle, to have the ability to recognize your needs and wants. You acknowledge that there are limits imposed on you by the group, but you can be happy with the place you are in. You are not miserable or anxious or too worried. You have accepted who you are at this time in your life. You have a good foundation and the skills to improve from there.

Now that you understand the fundamentals of laying down new tracts and shifting the "Me vs. Group" credibility needle, let's examine self-esteem in more detail and ways to improve yours.

Self-worth

First, let's think about self-worth. This is the feeling of being a good person or a bad person. Counselors want us to love ourselves unconditionally. This is not possible. As I have said, the group has a lot of say in our self-worth. What *is* possible is to define the parts of self-worth and calculate them accurately. There are at least three components to self-worth. The first is our accomplishments. What have we done, and have we been successful?

The second is our labeled portrait. This involves labeling all of our characteristics that we use to identify ourselves, such as father, brother, son, chunky, bald-headed, doctor, etc. The third component is the biological makeup of your brain that has a baseline of good/bad. How much dopamine or oxytocin do you produce, or how big or reactive is your amygdala?

Part 1: Accomplishments

When you finish a project and get a positive reception, you experience happiness. You have accomplished something. Maybe you think of what you are feeling as pride, or maybe it is just happiness. Whatever you call it, it feels good. You would like to have more of that. However, when your self-esteem is low, you rarely experience that feeling. More often than not, you fail and feel lousy—or you don't even try, which is like failing. Even if you have brief success, it comes with no carryover. You felt good for a few minutes, and then it is done, and you're back to not feeling good because something else didn't go right.

I have some insight that I want to share with you, information that I have not read in any book yet. *We really suck at counting our accomplishments.*

I like to use a point system when I talk about accomplishments. If I succeed, I get 10 points. If I fail, I get minus 10 points. That seems reasonable, doesn't it?

But here is what most people do. They calculate success at 1 point or, worse, zero points.

Why zero? Easy. Because it was something they were *supposed* to do, it doesn't count as an achievement. If I beat a 5-year-old in basketball, I get no achievement points because I was *supposed* or *expected* to beat him. The same with bigger things. If I work an 8-hour shift, I get no points because I was supposed to work to make money for my family.

But when I fail, I give myself a minus 10 points. People beat themselves up mercilessly. How could I have been so stupid? How could I be so incompetent? How will I ever face people again? You know what I'm talking about. We have a tendency to evaluate things worse than others around us. A minus 10 sucks. I am reminded of a scene from the movie *Liar Liar*. Jim Carrey is in the bathroom, trying to find a way to avoid returning to the courtroom because he can't lie, and he will lose the case. So, he beats himself up. Not just a little, a lot. He chokes himself, he punches himself, he hits his head with the toilet seat. He comes out of the bathroom disheveled, bruised, and swollen. He has kicked his own ass. How many times have you felt like that or seen someone else who had done that to themselves (metaphorically speaking)?

Not only do we keep a lopsided score, scoring failures way out of proportion to successes, we don't even count or credit all of our accomplishments. As I stated before, this occurs because we feel they were *supposed/expected* to be done, so there is no joy in the achievement. But there is also a second reason. We take our accomplishments for granted. We don't even acknowledge they are an accomplishment. Getting a glass of water from the sink is not usually thought of as an accomplishment. We take it for granted. We take it for granted until the well pump doesn't work or there is a power outage, and, all of a sudden, there is no tap water. Then we temporarily see that getting water from the sink is a big deal. But once the pump is fixed or the power restored, we quickly go back to taking water from the sink for granted.

You are an organism. Biologically speaking, your job is to stay alive and to keep the people in your family alive. Give yourself points for that. Staying alive is a big accomplishment. When I wake up in the morning, I open my eyes in bed and give myself 10 points for being alive. I roll over, and my wife is still breathing—another 10 points. I get out of bed and pour some water in a cup from the faucet—10 points for finding water. I go out to the kitchen and fix a bowl of cereal—10 points for finding food. I walk out back to eat the cereal and look at my house—add another 10 points for having a safe place. I start out the day with 50 self-esteem points. *Woohoo!* I get 50 points every day that I wake up.

Why doesn't everyone else take advantage of this? Because most people take those 5 things for granted. Returning to the movies, Tom Hanks is stranded on an island in *Castaway*. When he figures out how to make a shelter, when he figures out how to catch a fish, when he discovers how to make a fire and find a source of drinking water, he is jumping up and down, excited. He accomplished something. It was momentous. He did not take it for granted. We have to be the same way. When I wake up in the morning, I just scored 50 self-esteem points. You can, too. All you have to do is count them.

Now most people wake up and get no points because they take waking up for granted. Some even wake up and give themselves negative points because they are still here in this rat hole.

Let's see why my system is a way to feel more empowered. I wake up and get 50 points. During the day, someone gives me the opportunity to earn 20 points by doing something successfully. I am warned that, if I am not successful, I will lose 20 points. I look at the situation and say *Why not?* The worst that will happen is that I will end up with 30 points. But I could have 70 points. I go for it.

Someone else wakes up with minus 10 points. They don't feel good, but they are still putting in the effort to stay alive and hold up their responsibilities. They are given the opportunity to earn 20 points. Their thinking goes like this. If I succeed and get 20 points, that will give me good self-esteem. I like that idea. But if I fail, I will lose 20 points and be a minus 30. That risk is not worth taking. I will pass and stick with my minus 10.

Low self-esteem is self-perpetuating.

But you can change. You can keep score accurately. Give yourself a 10 for successes if you are going to give yourself a minus 10 for failures. Even more, you can count all your accomplishments. Take nothing for granted. And I mean *nothing*. Everything you do is an accomplishment. Staying alive is hard work. The things you do to stay alive are worthy of celebration.

I have done the math on my patients. You cannot have a negative score if you count accurately. It is not possible. If you count your successes equal to your failures, and you count all your successes, you will always be positive. Accomplishments make you feel good. Take credit for all you do. Feeling good is the reward.

2. Labeled portrait

Let's look at our labeled portrait and the "Me vs. Group" credibility meter.

We all have a mental portrait of ourselves, a picture of what we look like in general and a brief list of our major characteristics. This image is constantly changing. If I work out for six months and get thinner and more muscular, my picture changes. If I get skin cancer and my left ear is partially removed, the picture changes again. Interestingly, I have decided the reason decade birthdays are so notorious is because we change our portrait picture at that juncture. I am no longer in my twenties when I reach thirty. I am no longer in my fifties when I reach sixty. Usually, the portrait is not as flattering as you age, and, so, a decade birthday is where we mark our decline—then, set a fixed hold on our portrait for another 10 years.

What does this portrait have to do with the "Me vs. Group" credibility meter?

Let's look at this portrait with more detail. I have a rough picture of myself. I can look in the mirror or look at a photograph that includes me. I can identify my features well enough to know it is me and not someone else. But in my head, there is also a bunch of labels attached to my portrait. I am a man, a husband, a father, a son, a brother, a doctor, a teacher, an author, a basketball player, a karaoke singer, an exerciser, a brown-eyed person who is hard-working and smart, a reader, someone with a shaved head, a little overweight, and so on. There are lots of labels I can use to describe myself. Each label is assigned a score. Some are plus 10, some are minus 10, and some are neutral.

Where does that score come from?

It comes from some combination of "Me vs. Group" credibility. The group may think that being overweight is bad and give it negative points. It might think hard-working is good and give it plus 10 points. I can have my own scoring system. That is one of the freedoms we have in this country. The group might think my karaoke skills are a minus 10, but I think they are a plus 10. These scores are changeable. In 1900, being a marijuana smoker was a plus or, at worst, neutral. In 2000, a marijuana smoker was so negative that being slapped with that label could bring you jail time. Now, in 2021 in Maryland, a marijuana smoker is a plus as long as you have a government-issued card.

I can also change what I give high scores to. When I was in my teens and looking for a girlfriend, she had to be pretty. Now in my 50s, if I were looking for a girlfriend, she would have to be smart and hard-working. (That is not to imply anything about my wife's prettiness. Don't go there.)

So, going back to the portrait, I will give you an exercise that I give my patients. Draw a picture of yourself, and add as many labels as you can think of. Most people start dividing up good and bad labels. I'm hard-working—that is good. I am overweight—that is bad. I exercise, which is good; I watch TV too much, which is bad. I found that most labels are close to neutral. I have brown eyes. I shave my head. I drive a car.

In assigning labels, people fall into the same trap they did with achievements. They don't keep score accurately. A plus trait is a 1 or a zero value while a negative trait is a minus 10. The minus traits are put up in flashing neon lights for all to see (or hidden in a deep recess at quite a cost). When I was working with a patient with low self-esteem, she brought me her labeled portrait. She had 10 negative traits and 4 positive ones. We went through the list. She put being shy as a negative trait. I asked her where she got that score from. Clearly, she thought of it as negative, but I certainly did not. She was overweight. She drank alcohol to excess. She then put being a mother in the negative category. She told me she wasn't a good mother because she drank too much alcohol. I asked how her children were doing. She told me they were successful adults. She had fed them, nurtured them, taken them to school, put Band-Aids on their cuts. I decided she was a good mom who could have been better. When we did the final appraisal, there were 10 good traits and 4 bad ones. And the 4 bad ones could be changed. She could stop drinking; she could lose weight. When we tallied her overall score, it was 100 good and 40 bad, for a plus 60. Just as with achievements, there is no way to be negative on this scale. It is not possible.

Sometimes you have to adjust the meter. If you have pushed your needle all the way over to "Group," then you are left with the group's determination and none of your input. You need to move the needle back toward "Me" at least a little bit. Thanks to people pushing their needle, we have gone from seeing being gay as bad and something to hide and be ashamed of to seeing being gay as a plus that is celebrated with parades.

3. Brain chemistry

The third component that contributes to self-esteem is brain chemistry. This is something you are born with. It comes from your genes. In the past, it was not adjustable, but scientists now have better knowledge of how the brain works and have developed tools to make some changes. Medication can change the chemical balance in your brain and make you feel better, but that is a discussion beyond the scope of this book. This is an individual decision between your doctor and you. Nonetheless, I want you to know that your genes, your brain chemistry, does play a role in self-worth/self-esteem and that it is adjustable.

Let's talk about self-respect.

Self-respect is intertwined with the process of living. The process is defined by how you get to your achievements or your labeled portrait. You can't always be right or good. No one is. But you can have a process that takes you to the right answer more often. You can tweak the process if it goes off the rails, so that the next time, it works better. Knowing that you have a process and honing the process are accomplishments in and of themselves. The process insulates you if something goes wrong. It prevents your self-worth from taking a full hit by ensuring that nothing is a full failure.

A sports analogy might help with understanding this. If you are a batter in the Majors—I'll even make you a future Hall of Famer—you go to spring training, and you practice with a pitcher or a machine for hours a day. You build up your endurance with cardio exercises. You build up your strength with weightlifting. You watch videos of your swing with your coach to identify flaws, and you talk to your teammates about the opposing pitcher's tendencies. You have a process. You get to the plate, and two-thirds of the time, 66 out of 100 times, you don't get a hit. Your goal was to get a hit, and two-thirds of the time, you don't. But you are a future Hall of Famer because 33 percent of the time, you *do* get a hit, and 33 percent is *good* in BaseballWorld. Your process is effective.

Even more, you can tweak the process. You can lift more weights (or less). You can watch videos with a different coach. You can wear glasses or get better at identifying the curveball. Regardless, your self-respect is good because you have a good process, and that is an achievement.

Sitting on the opposite end of the spectrum is low self-respect. In this day and age, most people don't think they should be smoking. When I see a new patient, I ask them if they smoke. If they are smokers, 90 percent of the time they bow their heads in shame and answer, "Yes, I do smoke." They think smoking is wrong, but they do it anyway. By definition, this leads to low self-respect. They are engaged in an activity they don't think they should be engaged in. When a smoker stops smoking, they gain self-respect because they are now living their life the way they think they should.

If I have a friend making a lot of money in business, I respect him for his success. If I find out he is stealing money from his employees, my respect goes down because I don't think he is acquiring money in the right way. This is the same concept we use for ourselves. We judge whether we are doing things the right way. If I am the batter hitting .333 because I work and prepare diligently, I have a lot of self-respect. If I am embezzling money from my boss, my self-respect should go down.

You can be a better employee or a better parent or a better spouse or a better leader. You can read books, talk to counselors, exercise, meditate, keep a journal, or whatever else occurs to you in your process of improvement. Self-improvement is an accomplishment that can boost your self-esteem even if, at the end, you are not successful. You can always go back and tweak the process for the next time. A favorite line of mine is that *You are not a failure until you stop trying to succeed.*

Self-efficacy

Self-efficacy is also part of self-esteem. This component is based on a future you. Self-efficacy, as I define it, is how well you think you will do at some future task. If I ask you to give a talk to a large group of people, how well do you think you will do? People with high self-efficacy predict they will do well. They might think that because they have given a talk before that was successful, or because they will work hard and practice until they are good at it, or because they are successful at other endeavors and believe that will translate into success with this one. People with low self-efficacy are the opposite. Their prediction will be one of failure or underperformance. Their history will negatively color their future endeavors and accomplishments. Poor self-efficacy can be a self-fulfilling loop. You think you will do poorly at a new task, and you either don't try and give up easily or you define your work as a failure.

So how do I change my self-esteem?

By reading this chapter, you now understand what self-esteem is and the components that form it. This will give us a way to find the tools to get better. We have already discussed self-worth and the importance of keeping an accurate score and making sure you count all your accomplishments. I had to stop asking patients to write down their successes so they could see how many there were. Why? Because they developed cramps in their hand from writing about so many accomplishments. *I woke up, ate, drank, my car started, I made it to work, I earned a paycheck, I answered the phone, I had control of my bladder and bowels, I made it home, I fell asleep.*

You accomplish a huge amount every day, so take credit for it. The same goes for your labeled portrait. Make a list of the labels that describe you and, if you feel inclined, categorize them into good, bad, and neutral. Give yourself 10 points if they are good labels. If they are bad labels, there are 3 things you need to explore. First, can you change them? If you are a smoker, can you stop? If you are overweight, can you diet and exercise to lose weight? Second, examine your "Me vs. Group" credibility meter. Maybe your meter is pointed too far to the group side. Why give that other person so much credibility? Your clothes may be just fine even if a couple of your classmates make fun of them. You know as much as they do; your credibility counts just as much as theirs. Third, you can change the group. This is by far the hardest action and the one that takes the most time. History has been reshaped by people who changed the group. Being gay or black in America was not a good label, and there was little you could do to change individually. Thanks to the strength and perseverance of individuals working toward a common goal, those identities are now more positive.

The last thing I want to talk about is how to change your Perspective Prism. This is the construct that holds your beliefs, facts, standards, emotions, and level of consciousness. Your self-esteem is at its center. We are working hard to change that, but there are dependent ideas that come out of your low self-esteem, and they create a circular logic. I have low self-esteem, so I believe I am not worthy. I believe I am not worthy, so I have low self-esteem. These loops are hard to break. They have formed neural ruts in our brain. They are behind quotes like this: *I'm a waste of time. Nothing I do is good enough. I deserve pain. I'll never be happy.*

When these ideas are in your prism, they color how you see things. If nothing you do is good enough, you will find fault with everything you do. If you think you will never be happy, then even a fleeting experience of happiness will bring little joy because you'll know it won't last long.

Sometimes you need to change the facts. You can make a list of your facts and beliefs linked to your self-esteem and then examine them as if you were a scientist. The ideal scientist makes observations and does experiments to verify the facts and theories that form the backbone of science. There is a process in place that can accommodate change. Newton gave way to Einstein. Earthcentric gave way to Suncentric. Darwin provided an alternative to God. The process can be slow and resistant, but it allows for cataclysmic changes when it is deemed worthy. You, too, can be a scientist. Take the time to examine some of your beliefs about yourself. See how much is true and factual. How much is provable? How much is conjecture? Do an experiment or two. You will probably need to share the results with a friend, a spouse, or a counselor since your prism may influence whether you perceive the information accurately. As an example, when I was writing this book, I spent a lot of time asking others if details and analogies were accurate or clear and understandable. It helps to get others' opinions.

Now you are armed with your positive scorecard of achievements, positive labeled portrait, and your heightened credibility. You will see the inaccuracy of some of your past beliefs about yourself. Break the circular logic that has led to your lowered self-esteem. Discard ideas that keep you down, and replace them with the ideas that keep you up and happy.

Now that you have read this chapter and understand self-esteem, let me know if you can think up any other techniques to improve your self-esteem. Give me your suggestions on my website TheLessStressDoc.com.

LET'S RECAP
Definition of Self-Esteem
Self-esteem is an individual's accumulated judgment of their own self-worth, self-respect, and self-efficacy. Self-worth is the answer to the question "Am I a good person or a bad person?" Self-respect is a measure of whether a person is doing things the right way. Self-efficacy is a confidence measurement linked to an individual's ability to accomplish a task in the future.

Human Skill: Self-awareness, concept of good and bad, Perception Prism

Side effects: Sadness, anger, self-hatred

Tools:

- Realize self-esteem is made up of three components: self-worth, self-respect, and self-efficacy.

- Self-worth is answering the question, "Am I a good person?"

- Self-respect is answering the question, "Am I doing things the right way?"

- Self-efficacy is answering the question, "How will I do with a future task?"

- Realize self-esteem is started as soon as you have awareness that you are different from the people around you. That means it starts before age one.

- Know that the people around you, when you are young, have a lot of credibility; so the influence on your self-esteem is great.

- Believe that self-esteem can be changed.

- Know what the 4 D's are: Deny, Deflect, Diminish, Dismiss

- Be aware that self-esteem can be a self-fulfilling prophecy

- Be a scientist, challenge your long-held view of yourself. Most likely the evidence will point to a person who should have good self-esteem if you keep score accurately.

- Score your self-worth accurately. Give yourself ten points for all your accomplishments if you are going to give yourself minus ten points for your failures.

- Make sure you count all your accomplishments.

- If you count your successes equal to your failures and you count all your successes, you will always be positive.

- Give yourself proper credit for your labeled portrait. Count all your good characteristics as a ten if you are going to give yourself a ten for a bad characteristic.

- You have the ability to alter your bad characteristics.

- Examine where you are on the spectrum of your "Me vs. Group" credibility meter, and make sure there is at least some input from you.

- Counseling and medication are an option.

Practice, practice, practice. The more times you think of your self-esteem in a good way, the more entrenched it will become. You will start a neural network, an anatomical tract, that will get thicker and more automatic.

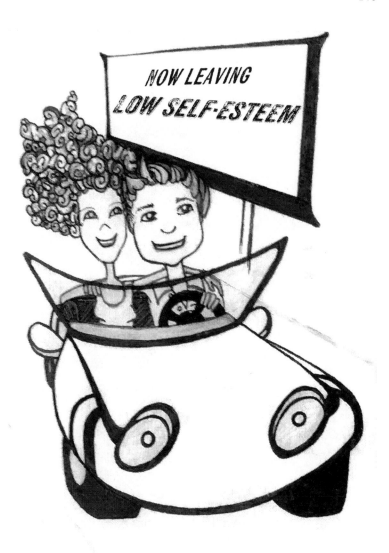

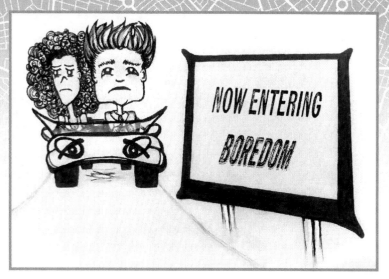

CHAPTER SIX

Boredom

Breaking Down Boredom

This chapter will define boredom in three ways: Lack of novelty, withdrawal syndrome, and thwarting your goal. You will be introduced to Joe, Billy, and Katie. I will discuss mindfulness and how that interplays with directed awareness. Ways to relieve boredom will include mindfulness, hope, repetition, and patience. There will be discussions about learning and viewing the opportunities in life. I will show you how to shift focus. Use human interaction to reduce boredom. Exercise and meditation are effective relievers. Finally, I will discuss imagination.

Definition of Boredom: Boredom has three separate conditions: One is a lack of novelty. One is a withdrawal syndrome from over-stimulation. And one is doing something that does not help you meet your goal.

Joe is a 34-year-old prisoner with bipolar disorder and Attention Deficit Hyperactivity Disorder (ADHD). He was convicted of attempted murder after he stabbed someone multiple times during a bar fight. He has been incarcerated for six years, but it has not gone well. He has been in multiple fights and landed in solitary confinement more than once. He hates solitary confinement. It is a punishment that far outweighs working on a chain gang in 30-degree weather or being punched in the face during one of his fights. As soon as the door closes on his solitary jail cell, Joe starts having a panic attack. He doesn't know how he is going to get through his time because it never seems to end. There is nothing to do. There is no one to talk to or fight with. There are only four walls, a small window, a metal cot, and his thoughts. His thoughts race through scenes, one after the other, with no coherence. Memories, fantasies, reality, his last fight, the warden, his girlfriend, his son. A minute has elapsed. Now he has 13 more days, 23 hours, and 59 minutes left to go.

Billy is a 9-year-old boy who lives in suburban DC. His parents work and make pretty good money. Billy has never wanted for anything. It is Saturday morning, and he has nothing to do. He is stuck at his grandparents' house because his parents have gone out of town for two weeks. He isn't allowed to bring his PlayStation because his grandparents think he should go outside and play. They are such old farts. He could watch TV, but they don't have cable, so he would have to watch some lame cartoon. There is a basketball court out back, but he doesn't want to play by himself. He is pretty good at reading, but there is nothing good to read here. They have toys to play with, but they are old and used, and they're not his toys. Who wants to play with them? His granddad suggested learning to play chess. Boring. His grandmother asked if he wanted to learn to bake bread. Seriously, he would rather watch the golf match that granddad has on, and he would rather die than watch golf. OMG. He has 13 more days of this to endure.

Katie is a 17-year-old junior in high school. She wants to be a nurse, so why is she sitting in a physics class? Who cares about vectors and the formula for velocity? What does this have to do with being a nurse? The physics teacher drones on and on—could he be any more boring? It is 5 minutes into class, and Katie has 40 minutes still to go. She is convinced she will die before the bell sounds.

These three scenarios are different, but they all describe a different facet of boredom. Let me get this straight right out front. For humans, boredom is one of the worst stresses there is. If you have a normal brain/mind, boredom is so bad you will do a lot of crazy things to stop it. I remember riding through an outdoor-mall parking lot in a pickup truck with my 16-year-old buddies, hour after hour, hoping something would happen that would stop the horrible boredom.

Low Input

Boredom can be the state of mind that occurs when there is no or little stimulation to the brain/mind. Joe in solitary confinement is an example of that. For two weeks he has no new stimulation to his brain. Solitary confinement has been known to do bad things to people. Boredom is so bad that, when someone is already being punished with a prison term, we use boredom to punish them even more. How bad can boredom be? BAD. Prisoners hate solitary confinement and will alter their behavior to avoid it.

Lack of stimulation is distressing to humans. The human organism has made behaviors that are essential to our survival pleasant. Eating, breathing, moving, sex, and being around others are pleasant and necessary for our survival. So is dealing with new environments, be they physical, psychological, or social. We need to be able to survive in many situations. Because of that, we've made novelty, and its emotional counterpart, curiosity, pleasant experiences. Lack of novelty, a true lack of novelty, is very unpleasant. Just as being hungry or horny are unpleasant urges, they spur us to alleviate them. Boredom pushes us to bring in novelty or to stimulate our curiosity. And we are willing to go to great lengths to do this.

If lack of novelty and lack of curiosity constitute boredom, is it any wonder that humans from the dawn of time have used sensory-altering drugs? What better way to get through a low-novelty day than by taking some drug that alters your senses and makes everything look different?

Don't get me wrong—the opposite of boredom is no fun, either. People can be overstimulated. But overstimulation doesn't engender the same persistent need as the urgency to alleviate boredom. You can dislike it when too much is going on, but you can more easily dampen down the overstimulation: you can close your eyes or go to a different room or outside. There are any number of techniques to decrease stimulation. But humans have few skills to counter boredom, to fix it when not enough is going on.

Humans do get used to a certain level of stimulation. A farmer in a small Appalachian town gets used to a lower level of stimulation than a stockbroker in New York City. But they both need some stimulation, some change, some novelty to make it through their existence. The novelty can be predictable. Working the farm during the sunlight, eating dinner at home, and sleeping in a feather bed. Church on Sunday. And once in a while, listening to bluegrass music on your neighbor's back porch on Saturday night. In most areas, weather provides novelty and becomes a topic of conversation that anyone can talk about. Novelty doesn't have to be something entirely new. It can be as small as a change from one setting to another. Some people are content to live their whole life doing one job, married to one person, and living in the same house. They are not bored. But if you put that same person in solitary confinement, removing all change, it wouldn't be long for that farmer to become distressed beyond consoling.

The other important factor in under-stimulation is age. Many books I've read support this idea. Again, this is a survival skill. When a human is young, curiosity is important. A human has to be exposed to a lot of different objects and activities to ensure survival. The more curiosity, the more exposure. The less curiosity, the less exposure, and the lower chance of survival. Once you have experienced enough of your environment, curiosity carries less importance for survival. That's why younger humans are more curious and seek more novelty than older humans. Humans don't lose their capacity for curiosity as they age, but it becomes a weaker drive. It becomes more associated with ensuring that there is no lurking danger around the corner. Curiosity, when you're young, pushes you to try something new for the sake of trying something new. Even so, young humans are way more likely to be bored than older humans.

The level of stimulation that is comfortable is different in every person. In general, young people want more stimulation, more novelty, and less routine. Older people want less novelty and more routine. As I'm writing this, I can see you shake your head. I'm not trying to say that older humans aren't curious or don't enjoy a new book or movie or learning a new skill. I'm saying that curiosity is a more powerful driver of young people's behavior. Older humans have more patience and greater ability to regulate the level of novelty in their environment. Young humans do not; their raw curiosity is more pressing.

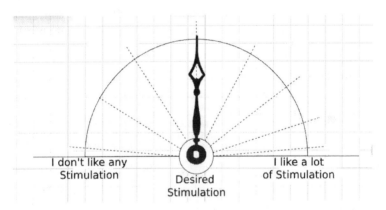

Every person has an individualized spot on the curve of desired stimulation. There is a range where they are content and happy. They also have a spot where they are under-stimulated and bored and a spot where they are over-stimulated. Novelty is a sweet spot that not only is different for everyone, but it also changes during your lifetime. It is one of the factors that attracts us to others. If you feel under-stimulated in your environment, you might seek out someone who takes more chances and is more outrageous.

If you are over-stimulated, you might seek out someone who is quiet and reserved, happy to stay home and watch a movie that you have seen before.

There is one more thing I wanted to discuss about this definition of boredom: sensory deprivation. Imagine a person suspended in a tank of saltwater. No lights. No sounds. No touch. As little sensory input as possible. This is the ultimate scenario for under-stimulation. There is no novelty. There is boredom. Someone who is over-stimulated and looking for relief from their stresses might consider this saltwater experience, but they would be purposely choosing this, and it would last only for a specific—and, I'm sure, short—period of time. Then it ends. It's probably nice not to feel anything for a short period of time, especially if you have been over-stimulated for long stretches. But if someone *forced* you to do this, with no end in sight, it would be a disturbing experience.

Withdraw

Billy's despair at his grandparents' house falls under our second condition for boredom. Every parent has been faced with a Billy who is flopping on the couch, complaining that he is bored and that there is nothing to do. There might be a big-screen TV, countless books, sports equipment, arts and crafts, toys, neighbors, woods, bikes, skateboards, a trip to an amusement park planned for next week, and dinner due in an hour. But Billy is bored, with a capital B. This is not sensory deprivation. This is not lack of novelty. This is not a rut. This is not an environment where curiosity is absent. Yet everyone would call this boredom and understand what was meant.

Billy says he is bored. He has plenty of stimulation, plenty to be curious about, and plenty of novelty. There is no way he should be bored, yet he sits on the couch complaining. What is really happening is a withdrawal from over-stimulation. Stimulation corresponds to the level of adrenaline that we are used to. When the stimulation is reduced, the adrenaline level goes down. A physical withdrawal syndrome occurs in tandem with this drop in adrenaline. It is physiological. It is psychological. It is predictable.

This withdrawal sensation is uncomfortable, at best, and miserable at worst. Humans do not like this sensation and, just as with drug addiction, their behavior is directed toward making this feeling go away. Usually that involves doing something that stimulates the release of adrenaline. However (and again like drug addiction), it takes more and more stimulation to get the desired effect.

This need for adrenaline is not limited to the individual. Entire group settings revolve around it. I would even go as far as saying our country's culture is addicted to adrenaline. We are in an adrenaline stress-reducing loop. We crave situations that will release adrenaline—amusement parks with bigger and faster roller coasters, bungee jumping, daredevil stunts, and sporting events in which winning is everything and losing is horrible. More-realistic video games that simulate war. Movies that are so vivid that it is hard to distinguish them from reality. We want more and more and more stimulation.

There are even careers packed with stimulation. Think of the ambulance crew, the emergency-room staff, the work of a stock-market trader.

We crave the stimulation and consequent adrenaline rush. When there is a drop in the level we are used to, we feel bored. The only antidote is bigger and faster and scarier and more important activities and events, until we overwhelm ourselves with stress.

Let's send our Appalachian farmer to New York. A person used to the slow pace of rural life would quickly get overwhelmed by the traffic, the crowds of people, the fast speech, the rushing, the noises, the size of the buildings. He might enjoy it for a day or two, but it wouldn't be long before he starts to crave his farm again. Back at home, he could take a deep breath and enjoy the routine and pace of his life. If going home wasn't an option, and he had to stay in New York, he would adjust to the pace and reset his "normal" on the novelty curve, or he would be miserably over-stimulated.

Now let's take that stockbroker in New York City and send him to an Appalachian farm. He would be moving too fast, speaking too fast, wondering why there is only one restaurant, one grocery store, and a Dollar General store to buy clothes. The largest building is the county courthouse. Everyone knows everyone, and there is no hiding. He feels uncomfortable. He is anxious. He doesn't know what to do next because there is so little to do. There is no one to talk to who understands his dilemma, because the local people can't believe he likes living in New York. He is withdrawing from the stimulation of New York.

Like the farmer, two options stand ahead of this stockbroker. He can withdraw and reset his spot on the novelty curve, slowing down and learning to enjoy the local pace. He can develop more deeply connected relationships with the few people who live nearby and learn to look forward to when the yearly carnival comes to town. Or he can remain permanently bored, waiting for the first chance to go back to New York. He will be miserable until he opts for one of those paths.

In these two examples, if the farmer becomes accustomed to New York, or the stockbroker gets used to Appalachia, and they reset their sweet spot on the novelty curve but then return to their respective homes, the farmer will be bored, and the stockbroker will be overwhelmed until they can readjust.

I watched *The Hurt Locker*, a movie about a soldier who defused bombs. It was extremely nerve-wracking work. But he loved it. When his tour was finally over, he returned home to his wife and kid. After a nice reunion with his loving family, he resumed a life with no more worries about bombs exploding or dying suddenly. But the next scene in the movie finds the soldier in the grocery store deciding between corn flakes or Cheerios. It didn't take long for him to become bored. He reupped in the military and went back to the more-stimulating war scene.

If boredom is an adrenaline withdrawal, how do people fix that? They increase the stimulation or push the adrenaline. Kids look for a more-stimulating video game or a more-realistic movie. They play or watch a sport and up the stakes so that the payoff of winning is greater. They do anything to stop the feeling of withdrawal that we have labeled *boredom*.

Doesn't this sound like a chemical addiction? I agree. If someone is taking opioids or benzodiazepines, their body gets used to the current dose and needs more to get the same reaction. If the person stops taking the chemical, there is a significant withdrawal reaction. So, then the person takes more and more of their drug in search of the feel-good result. But now, even at high doses, they might not achieve that. Still, at least they are avoiding the horrible withdrawal feelings that come with not having it at all. Boredom carries a lot of parallels to chemical addiction and adrenaline stimulation.

Roadblock to Goals

Katie, the 17-year-old student, personifies our third form of boredom: doing something that does not take you to your goal. Katie has a specific goal to become a nurse. There are classes she needs to accomplish that. When she is in classes that don't carry her toward her goal, frustration occurs, and boredom sets in. She doesn't want to study physics. She doesn't see how it will help her become a nurse. When a person suffers from this type of boredom, they will fall asleep, daydream, procrastinate, complain, or avoid the situation. This form of boredom is uncomfortable and typically comes with low curiosity. After all, people don't want to spend a lot of energy on something that doesn't help them advance their goal. The longer the time spent on the unrewarding activity, the worse the boredom, and the greater the distress.

Now we know the three forms of boredom. One is the literal lack of stimulation. The body craves stimulation, which is why solitary confinement is the ultimate punishment for someone already in prison. The second form of boredom is the withdrawal of stimulation. When a person is used to a certain level of stimulation and it is taken away, boredom sets in. The third type of boredom comes from an activity that delays or separates a person from their desired goal. It's time to fix this problem of boredom.

What can be done to alleviate boredom?

There is actually a lot that can be done, once you understand what boredom is. I will share my mantra: better understanding, better tools, better results.

Let's explore the solutions to each form of boredom separately, realizing there will be some overlap.

Use mindfulness, which is control of your directed awareness. As I said earlier, a short period without stimulation can be therapeutic. However, longer stints can be painful and actually damaging to a person. The brain and mind require a certain amount of novelty, or they become permanently altered. Prisoners develop serious psychological problems from being in solitary confinement for too long.

For the solution to this type of boredom, I turn to monks. Many monks live with great deprivation. They don't talk for a year, they pray for hours and hours, they don't eat for days at a time. Their level of stimulation could be close to zero, and, yet, they see this deprivation as a way to grow. I don't know why they choose this, but the way they avoid boredom is through mindfulness, which I would describe as *gaining control of your directed awareness*.

The more control you have of your directed awareness, the more stimulation you have access to. Your memory is made up of many—maybe millions—of scenes and bits of information. You have multiple emotions that you can call forth at will. (This is an actor's skill.) If faced with a lack of external stimulation, you turn to your inner memories and facts for the stimulation your brain/mind needs. In doing this, you learn that you really have a lot of control. You can go slow or fast, you can bring up specific memories, or you can learn to appreciate the random memories that surface without stimulation. You can learn to call forth an emotion at your command. When you get better at controlling your directed awareness, you can stop emotions and memories from flooding your awareness while gaining access to more of your memories and emotions. The reduced or nonexistent external stimulation allows your directed awareness to retrieve past information more easily; it allows access to information that was hidden or clouded by the external world. The availability of new information could lead to insights that might change your life or alter your perspective on your current life. Maybe that is why monks choose lives of deprivation.

Keep hope alive. Hope comes from envisioning the future and seeing a better tomorrow. A person with hope can tolerate a lot of pain or discomfort because they believe it will end at some point. I see this in my patients who have pain. If it is short-term pain, and/or the patient believes the pain will go away, the patient is willing to tolerate a great deal of pain and will require much less pain medication. But if a patient believes the pain will never go away, they have less ability to handle the pain without medication. Hope keeps people from committing suicide. When a person thinks things will never get better, what is the point to staying alive? The person with hope believes it will get better, and, because of that, there are lots of reasons to persevere. Hope is critical to surviving a low-to-no stimulation environment.

Repetition helps. The movie *Papillon* stars Steve McQueen and Dustin Hoffman. McQueen's character was in prison but continued to get in trouble and spent weeks in solitary confinement. His solution was repetition. He would walk around his cell, counting his steps each time. He developed a routine and repeated it over and over. This routine kept him stimulated and kept his brain from being damaged. We see this in zoo animals when they pace a specific pattern. Obsessive-Compulsive Disorder (OCD) is a form of stress reduction. The routine could be a physical behavior or a mental pattern. They are giving the brain what it craves—stimulation. Cigarette smoking and prayer with rosary beads involve repetitive actions. They relieve stress.

Patience is necessary. Now let's turn our attention to the form of boredom in which there is a withdrawal of stimulation. Again, there are several methods to reduce the discomfort of this withdrawal. The most important is the recognition that this feeling or discomfort will go away with time. People withdrawing from alcohol and heroin know it will stop and that their body and brain will go back to normal. Boredom goes away after time. Patience is the first step. Be patient, and your brain/mind will adjust to the new, lower level of stimulation.

I would not recommend increasing the stimulation. Like heroin and alcohol addiction, as you build up tolerance, it takes more and more stimulation to get the same effect. This is why no matter how much stimulation we give our kids, they get bored. Eventually they build up a tolerance to adrenaline.

Use mindfulness or directed awareness. Mindfulness allows us to pick and choose where our awareness is focused. When there is withdrawal from stimulation, you can use mindfulness or directed awareness to change the focus from macro to micro or micro to macro, or present to past or past to future. If I am bored watching TV, I can direct my awareness to a book, or I can learn a new skill or focus on exercise. I get to choose where my mind finds stimulation to alleviate the feeling of boredom. Control comes from making choices, and this gives you control. Control might be illusory, but the more I sense I am in control, the less anxious and the better I feel. I feel empowered when I can control my focus, and this power will reduce the withdrawal symptoms.

Changing levels of focus or tenses—from present to future, for example—I can make a difference. I can focus on my hand and notice the anatomy and the interplay of fingers, hands, and wrists. Or I can go deeper and tap the internet to see how the blood vessels and nerves and ligaments interact. Or I can go deeper still to the cellular or the atomic level. On the other hand, I might choose the big picture, visualizing how I collaborate with other humans, how societies work, or how Earth fits into the universe. I can change tense, looking back to my past or into the past of our country or culture—or I can look forward to the future and try to predict where I will be in one day, one month, one year, or one decade. You get the idea. You can control what you focus on, and changing the focus will reduce the feeling of boredom.

Learn something new. Let's revisit our nursing student. Katie is bored because she doesn't know why she is taking a physics class. She doesn't understand physics and can't see how this applies to nursing. What if, instead of seeing physics as a boring roadblock, she sees it as a challenge? Challenging herself to learn something new might begin to alleviate her boredom. I remember my son and I watching a cricket game on TV while visiting London. Neither of us knew anything about cricket, and, consequently, we might have been very bored except that we decided to try to learn the rules. We watched the crowd and reacted when they did. We looked for patterns in the action. We watched for an hour and enjoyed ourselves. We didn't become avid cricket fans, but we weren't bored, and, in fact, we gained a newfound appreciation for cricket.

When you come at something as a challenge, it gives you the opportunity to succeed. And, as you'll recall, success leads to improved self-esteem and a good feeling. It gives you the confidence and motivation to take on something new in the future.

Look for opportunity. Instead of seeing physics as an obstacle, Katie could try to see it as an opportunity to expand her knowledge. Knowledge is power. The more knowledge you have, the more power you have. Knowledge might be used now, or it might be used in the future. Maybe as a nurse, Katie will find herself taking care of a patient who is a physicist, and that patient might appreciate even her rudimentary knowledge of physics. That could make the patient feel more comfortable as he recuperates from an operation. I had this experience. I was taking care of a mathematics professor who had just had a stroke. I didn't know a lot about math, but I knew some things, and it made him feel better to talk to someone who could appreciate the knowledge. In talking about math, he felt that he hadn't lost everything with his stroke. The more I learn, the more empathetic I can be. I can carry on a conversation with a mathematics professor, a doctor, a teacher, a construction worker, a day-care provider, or even a pilot because I have learned information over my years that enables me to communicate with people on their level and on their favorite topics.

Shift the focus. If I find myself watching a TV show I don't like or is boring, I will shift my focus. Instead of actually watching the show, I will put myself in the director's chair and wonder why she picked that angle to show the kiss. I will watch the actor and discover why I don't believe his anger or compare him to a better actor who is more believable. I will think about the differences between the two of them. Changing focus like this stops boredom because it requires redirecting my thought, effort, learning, or analysis. Try it.

Sensory-altering chemicals. There are plenty of legal chemicals that can change perception and add novelty to your environment. Caffeine, sugar, teas, espresso, alcohol, etc. These chemicals alter perception in some way. Some offer big changes, and some offer small changes. I do counsel caution. These chemicals all have benefits, but they also have side effects. Alcohol is one in particular. It is a drug that can make a boring situation more tolerable, but you have to use the right dose and frequency. Addictions (stress-reducing loops) can develop. Tolerance and withdrawal can lead to more problems than boredom. Side effects can outweigh the risks. But, if used judiciously, these chemicals can be useful.

Human interaction relieves boredom. When I was a teenager riding around in a parking lot, I was with friends. Humans enjoy being around other humans. Talking to someone else can be enough to relieve boredom. In our current society, phones and computers have allowed us to talk to people anywhere in the world. These technologies increase the amount of people we can communicate with. They have also made human interaction safer in some ways, because if I don't like or trust what you have to say, I can just hang up or sign off. I can have a relationship with someone in Iceland or Thailand. There is always going to be someone, somewhere in the world with similar thoughts and feelings to mine. I just have to find them.

Physical exercise is a boredom buster. When you're in physical motion, it takes your brain's and mind's full focus so that you don't fall, trip, or collide with something. Being physically tired, too, can reduce your brain's need for stimulation. When you are tired from physical exertion, your brain is healing and repairing what you just did to your body by running for a mile, biking through your neighborhood, or shooting basketball with friends.

Use meditation to slow down. While physical activity can counteract boredom, so, too, can slowing down. With meditation, you slow everything down, focus on your breathing, and try to rid your muscles of energy. Meditation helps you learn to control your tone, your thoughts, your breathing, and your emotions by focusing on these concepts.

Tap your imagination. Humans are amazing creatures. Among our mind's great skills is imagination. By using concepts and words, we can rearrange reality. Instead of a father with two eyes and two ears, why not imagine a father with no ears and four pairs of eyes. Instead of a car, why not envision a rocket-propelled vehicle with no wheels that floats on a cushion of air. What would the world be like with cars that didn't have wheels? No need for roads anymore. Interesting. Imagination can take you wherever you would like to go and change your reality to your liking. Wouldn't it be fascinating to be in J.K. Rowling's imagination as she creates Hogwarts, Harry Potter, and the wizarding world? It's OK to use other people's imagination, too. Read a book, watch a movie, talk to friends.

Now that you have read this chapter and understand boredom, let me know if you can think up any more techniques for reducing boredom. Give me your suggestions on my website, TheLessStressDoc.com.

LET'S RECAP
Definition of Boredom
Boredom has three separate conditions. One is a lack of novelty. One is a withdrawal symptom from over-stimulation. And one is doing something that does not help you meet your goal.

Human Skill: Curiosity
Side effect: Psychological pain, apathy, psychosis
Tools:

- Boredom as under-stimulation.

  - Stimulate your curiosity, and act on it.

  - Find new challenges or learn new skills.

  - Learn more details about a topic you already know a lot about.

  - Keep up hope that your situation will improve.

  - Repetition.

- Boredom as withdrawl

  - Be patient—the worst symptoms of boredom will go away with time. Boredom is not lethal.

  - Adjust the sweet spot of novelty to fit your environment: In a fast-paced environment, speed up. In a slow-paced environment, slow down.

  - Use mindfulness to gain control of your directed awareness.

  - Use mindfulness to shift your focus. From micro to macro, from past to future, from outer to inner.

- Boredom as a roadblock to your goal.

  - Learn something new that might not apply now but will come in handy in a later setting.

  - Physical Exercise.

- ~ Meditation.

- ~ Use legal chemicals to provide novelty.

- ~ Use human interaction to your benefit

- ~ Use your imagination—or someone else's, in the form of a book or movie.

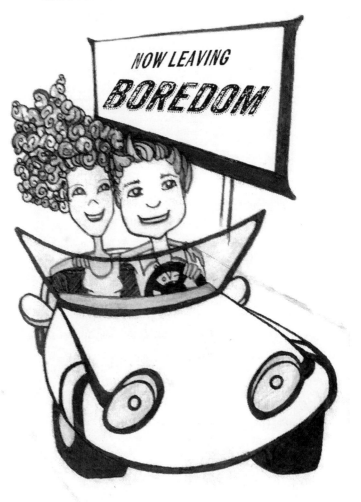

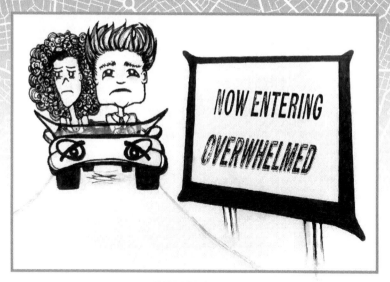

CHAPTER SEVEN

Overwhelmed

Are You Feeling Trapped, With No Way Out?

I will define what being overwhelmed means. I will introduce Bridgette as an example. I will show you why, when people get overwhelmed, they get mislabeled as depressed. Being overwhelmed can result from too many stresses or one big stress. Your response to stress can be categorized as a low reactor or high reactor. I will show a way to get out from feeling overwhelmed with some very specific tools, such as The Shoe Box, The Adjustable Map, Transformational Vocabulary, and others.

Definition of Overwhelmed: Being overwhelmed is a state in which there are too many issues that require attention or one much-too-big one. It is based on fear and sadness. It is often mislabeled as depression. It can occur in other animals but is way more likely in humans, because humans have so many more sources of stress.

*B*ridgette *just emerged from the courtroom.* The judge had agreed to grant the divorce, but the child support and visitation rights still needed to be ironed out. Matt is such a pain in the ass. The judge couldn't see how much he was lying and hiding. The judge didn't get to see the verbal abuse he inflicted on Bridgette. How many times had she had been told she was a piece of crap? Now Bridgette was free. Well, "free" might be too strong a word. She had to work two jobs to make enough money to pay her bills. She had to find child care for her three kids. She couldn't sleep at night, so she spent most of her waking hours feeling tired. Her youngest child had asthma and simply being in the midnight air might result in a trip the ER at any given time. Her parents were as helpful as they could be, but they lived four hours away. Matt had moved out months ago, which made living in the house more pleasant, but it also meant she had to repair whatever went wrong or hire someone cheap enough that she could afford.

Bridgette woke up every morning realizing what an insurmountable task she faced. Each day brought more problems and hassles. There was no end in sight. She didn't know how she was going to make it through today.

Unfortunately, I hear stories like Bridgette's way too often. There are numerous variations, but the underlying theme is constant: *There are too many problems at one time for me to face, and I can no longer cope.* This is the stress of being overwhelmed. It is interesting that, when I tell someone they are overwhelmed, their body language changes. The patient feels that one word— *overwhelmed*—describes their whole life. There is recognition: *That is exactly how I feel.* For a brief moment, they know that someone understands them—and then the reality of their situation regains its chokehold. Tears stream down their face because they have so many issues and no clue how to manage them all.

I've been there. I was told I was depressed. Is that the same as being overwhelmed?

Being overwhelmed has often been mislabeled as depression. Patients diagnosed with depression have a lot of physical and psychological symptoms. They stop eating, or they can't stop eating. They hardly sleep, or they sleep too much. They spend their day in a mental fog. Their thinking is disorganized, so they don't accomplish much on any given day. They are tired. They can't enjoy themselves because the pressure is immense. Responsibility is weighing them down.

Sometimes they will spend the whole day in their room. Their boss will complain that they are forgetful, not accomplishing enough, or distracted. This adds to the worries they already have and makes the patient feel even more overwhelmed. The patient has an inordinate amount of fear with anger, guilt, regret, and frustration mixed in. Patients feel like they are on a roller coaster. Their emotions come and go without any control. But the predominant emotion is sadness. There is a resignation that there is no way out. Most doctors label a patient with these symptoms as being depressed. They tell their patient that this comes from a chemical imbalance, and, if they just take this pill every day, they will feel better within the month. Go see a therapist. Next patient.

I strenuously disagree with this assessment. Maybe that's why you and I are working here together. The average doctor isn't helping solve your problems as much as he/she is covering them up.

Doctors aren't stupid—they are just doing what they have been taught to do: put together a group of symptoms, label the condition, and treat it, based on available studies. The problem goes back to what doctors are being taught. Depression is considered a chemical imbalance. If you believe that, then it makes sense to take a pill (chemical) to change the balance to a more favorable place. But is it really an imbalance? What is the evidence? This is where the mistake lies. All studies on depression medications are conducted on rats. Researchers make a rat depressed then they give it a chemical they know affects the chemistry of the brain. Then, they observe its effects. With rats, they can dissect the brain and do studies about the chemistry that could never be done on humans. Armed with the information that a depressed rat does better on this medication, they apply the finding to humans. They make sure the medicine is safe and then try it out on people who meet the criteria for depression. Frequently, those people *do* feel better. The scientist then makes a leap of logic: *This patient feels depressed; they take a medicine that affects some chemical transmitter in the brain; they feel better; therefore, they have a chemical imbalance, and, as a consequence, all patients with depression should be treated with a chemical (medicine) for their chemical imbalance.*

There are several fatal flaws in this thinking. First, the last time I checked, humans are not rats. They may have similarities in their brain structure, but humans are not rats. Therefore, any study on the brain that is run on rats cannot be that accurate. Humans have a mind, and rats do not. Humans have a future, and rats do not. Humans have choice and the ability not to do what their brain has been trained to do, and rats do not. Humans have words and concepts, and rats do not.

Secondly, since doctors really have no idea what depression is except within a rat model, they try all different sorts of chemicals that cause all kinds of changes in the brain. There are no fewer than five different classes of chemicals that can be altered and will have a positive impact on depression. That alone is an indication that doctors don't really understand the cause of depression. A doctor sees a study, identifies a group of patients with the symptoms of depression, gives them a medication that alters some known chemical transmitter in the brain, and then observes the effects. If the patient's symptoms improve, the erroneous assumption is made that the patient must have lacked that chemical, that the chemical was out of balance in the patient, and that changing the balance cured the patient. A cause-and-effect conclusion is being made, but the error is that the conclusion is being made based on assumptions from rat research.

Let's say the chemical-imbalance model is correct. If a person feels better after drinking alcohol, does that mean they are alcohol deficient? Am I curing their depression by giving them alcohol? If they drink alcohol, they might smile more, be more outgoing, or laugh at my karaoke version of "Doctor Love." Alcohol works very well as an antidepressant. But the problem comes when people use the wrong dose—usually too much. When that happens, the alcohol has an opposite effect. No one feels better.

I used an absurd example. If a person feels better on alcohol, no one decides they are alcohol deficient. But if I give you a serotonin reuptake inhibitor and it works, then I assume you are serotonin deficient. This works for norepinephrine, GABA, and a slew of other brain chemicals.

If patients really have a chemical imbalance, then adjusting their chemistry should fix the problem. It does not. I have treated a lot of depressed patients with medications, and, at best, they feel a little better. They still have a ton of problems, but the problems don't seem as big. Their mood is a little better. However, if some new problem comes along, these patients go right back to exhibiting their symptoms, despite increases in the dosage of the medication.

Doctors can go only on what they know. The experts all say that depression is a chemical imbalance, and that, by adjusting the chemistry with a pill, the patient will improve. So that's the route that doctors take.

I want to give you a new way to think about how doctors approach psychiatric problems. There is a book called the *DSM-5*. This book catalogues all the psychiatric illnesses. Each illness has a set of criteria for labeling a patient with any particular diagnosis. In essence, each illness is a box of symptoms. If you have enough of the symptoms in that box, you get the label on that box. Most patient have multiple symptoms when they seek help. The symptoms can overlap in the *DMS-5*; one symptom might be found in multiple boxes. Inattention might be Attention Deficit Disorder (ADD), or it might be depression. Inability to sleep could be bipolar disease, mania, or schizophrenia. Symptoms and signs are open to interpretation. A paranoid person might actually have someone after them, meaning their fear is normal.

And what about a person who fits in multiple boxes? A patient can be bipolar, depressed, have ADD, have substance-abuse disorder, be schizoaffective, or have borderline personality disorder, depending on how doctors interpret the same set of symptoms and a patient's behavior and feelings. Unlike diabetes, there is no blood test that tells you a person is depressed. It is all open to interpretation.

I want you to look at depression in a new way. I want to make a new box called "Overwhelmed." I want you to think of it as a syndrome. A syndrome is a bunch of symptoms and physical signs that doctors group together and label. A syndrome is a way to find a pattern that could lead to better understanding of what caused the problem to begin with—as well as a better way to treat it. So, what might cause depression syndrome? It could be a chemical imbalance. We have information that, by changing the chemistry of the brain, a person can feel better. But the vast majority of patients labeled with "Depression Syndrome" are not chemically imbalanced. (There *are* patients who *do* have a chemical imbalance and do very well with medicine and poorly without, but this is a minority of patients.) I think most patients are overwhelmed—living with more stress than they can handle. I believe Depression Syndrome is more accurately labeled "Overwhelmed Syndrome."

We have learned the sources of some of human stresses: worry, guilt, regret, low self-esteem, boredom. As I stated in the beginning of this book, humans are the most stressed organism that has ever existed on this planet. Our brain has brought us the greatest achievements, but that process comes with side effects. When these stresses accumulate, they can overwhelm our abilities to handle them. This leads to the symptoms that we have formerly described as "Depression" but which I want to re-label as "Being Overwhelmed." *Overwhelmed* is a more accurate reflection of what is actually taking place. Most importantly, it leads us to different and more beneficial treatments.

Being overwhelmed is a scary place. For someone used to feeling in control, being beyond your coping skills is like being in a place you have never been before. In a new country, the language is different, the food is different. Even the bathrooms are different. No one thing is overwhelming on its own, but when you put them all together, you don't even know where to start. You can't read your roadmap because the alphabet and language are unfamiliar.

Another analogy for being overwhelmed: Think of trying to pay a $500 doctor bill when you only have $300. You have some money but not enough. If a new bill for $5 comes in, it is devastating. You already lack the money to cover the first bill. I recently saw a patient who was in his 80s. He had enjoyed reasonably good health, he had been married for more than 60 years, he made sufficient money, his kids were successful adults, and he had always felt in control. But now his own health was failing, his wife was developing early dementia, his independence was being taken away, and his own mortality was staring him in the face. He was getting angry and upset at the least little thing. He was shaking his cane at his wife for not remembering an appointment. His kids were worried about him. In a word, he was *overwhelmed*. For him, it was frightening, because he had never been there before. He had no idea what to do or even how to describe what was going on.

When I labeled his condition as *overwhelmed*, he immediately understood. He did not want to be diagnosed as "Depressed."

He didn't feel sad. He wasn't staying in his room, contemplating suicide. People feel better when I say they are *overwhelmed*, as opposed to when they are told they are *depressed*. Overwhelmed is a more accurate description, and it carries a different fix. Medication is not going to be the only answer. Don't get me wrong: Medication can help, but it is not a cure. To get a cure, we have to have a better understanding of the underlying principles that brought the person to this place of being overwhelmed.

The basic model for humans with a brain and/or a mind is:

Stress ⟶ Stress Reducer ⟶ Less Stress

This is a broad statement, but it is the equation that underpins much of what we do. Stress can be physical, as when there is a hurricane or heat spell. The stress can be social, such as being shunned, or psychological, when there are feelings of low self-worth. It could be economic insecurity (not enough money), and so on. It can be lodged in the past, as with a traumatic event, or in the present, in the form of a mean boss, or in the future, like when you are worrying about what kind of world your two-year-old will live in. It can be local; a gunman is shooting people at a nearby gas station. Or it can be global; the oil supply is threatened by a boycott or a war. It could be a cosmic event where *God has forsaken me* or there are extraterrestrials and/or zombies threatening me. Humans have few boundaries when it comes to what they feel or view as stressful.

So how does a person get overwhelmed, if this is the basic premise?

It can occur in several ways. Some are obvious, and some are not as easily identified. At the most basic, it is simply too many stresses. In fact, this is the most common problem I see with patients. Someone will list every problem they have and add them all up into a big, giant ball of stress. When you have a lot of stressful things going on and lump them all together, you get overwhelmed. A person in this situation may actually start looking for *more* things to throw on top. They'll remember one other thing that is going to add to their ball of stress. I'm not sure why that occurs—if you are already stressed out, why look for more?—but it happens all the time.

Not everyone with a lot of stress gets overwhelmed. When you watch a war movie, there is a crazy amount of stress. People are trying everything they know to kill the soldier. He might not be safe with even his own buddies. Because of the increased stress, there may increased use of alcohol and other mind-altering substances. The soldier's buddy could be drunk and get mad at him—and he has an M16 rifle in his possession. Some people handle this situation, and others get overwhelmed. So the number of stressors is a factor but not the only one.

It is important to keep in mind that people react to stress along a physiological spectrum. Some people are on the high-re-actor end, while others are on the low-reactor end. I think this is a result of two factors. One, and probably most important, is genetic. I think high-reacting or low-reacting responses can be inherited. Your brain has been set up to have a danger response. It can have a big reaction to danger or a smaller one. If the brain is highly sensitive or highly responsive, you will have a big reac-tion—and vice versa.

The second component is your education. If your parents or close connections are high reactors, you will learn from them that that is how you are supposed to respond in a given situation. Or if your surrounding group are low reactors, you will learn to be less reactive. Of course, you also have some choice as to which person or group you use as your lead example.

Learning is important, but your DNA is more fundamental here. Most couples, I find, reflect an intersection of high and low reactors. Two high reactors won't last long, and two low reactors rarely get together. That means a child usually has some influence from both pathways.

Let's look at low reactors with few stressors first. Life is reasonably straightforward for them, and they operate within their comfort zone. The only time I see a low-reactor person in my office with psychological issues is when a huge catastrophic event occurs. It might be a self-inflicted problem, such as engaging in something illegal and getting caught, or it might be caused by someone in their immediate family having a huge crisis, or it could be an external event like a flood or hurricane. People who don't usually get overwhelmed can cross that threshold with a catastrophic event. Since this person never leaves their comfort zone, they have no experience in knowing how to handle overwhelming situations. This is where my elderly patient found himself.

The next category of patients is the low reactor with a lot of stressors. Low-reacting people can have a lot of stuff going on. I use soldiers as an example. At their military base, they are fine, but in the throes of a war zone, they can get overwhelmed. Someone is shooting at them. The rules that have guided their lives are no longer in effect. They find themselves doing things they would never do back home. In a military study during the Vietnam era, up to 90 percent of soldiers had some sort of addiction. The military was worried about what would happen when all those soldiers with addictions came home. Fortunately, their home environments were a lot less stressful, and most soldiers no longer needed chemical crutches. Still, I'm sure there was at least 20 percent who did not stop. I would bet that their environments were still very stressful, such as living in an inner city, being in a place where there were no jobs, or having to manage Post-Traumatic Stress Disorder (PTSD).

The two categories of patients I see frequently in the office are high reactors. These people react very strongly to the stressors they encounter. When there are few stressors, they can manage (although sometimes it's a struggle). But it doesn't take many stressors to overwhelm their coping skills. They are easily overwhelmed, not because they are weak or deficient, but because they react so strongly to their stressors. If every stress is a 10, how many stressors does it take before you have too many? It takes a lot to get their reactions down to a tolerable level. They have to use more powerful treatments and use them more frequently. These patients are at risk for addictions (Stress Reducer Loops is a concept I will detail in my upcoming book *New Outcomes*). If you give a high reactor a lot of stress, overwhelmed is the norm.

The fourth category, when a high reactor has a lot of stressors, it gets to be more than overwhelmed. There is also a category *beyond being overwhelmed*. I call this *Being Numb*. At that level, the person is not functional. They sit in their room and don't come out, or they rock, with a blank stare. This is a bad and dangerous place to be. This level of being overwhelmed requires more intensive intervention. It can be treated successfully but usually requires in-patient services and is beyond the scope of this book.

Here is an S-graph. The S-graph is what I use with patients to show the continuum of Being in Control to Overwhelmed to Numb.

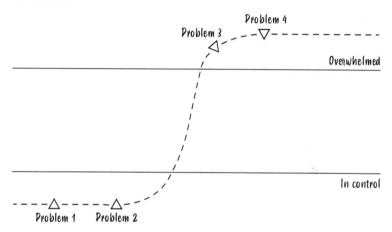

As you can see, with one or two problems, a person is under control and can handle the situation. But when a third or fourth problem is added, there is a steep rise, which is how it got its name, "S curve." This is when the patient feels overwhelmed. The curve is steep, because one day the person can feel in control, and the next day or next hour, when a new problem is added, the feeling of being overwhelmed occurs. The same S curve is seen when someone gets even more stress and ends up in the *Numb* category. I use this graph a lot with patients. It helps them to visualize what is going on. It makes being overwhelmed a little less scary. It shows them that, even though it took only one problem to feel overwhelmed, it will take the elimination of only one problem to feel back in control.

Being overwhelmed becomes one of the problems on the graph line. It gets added to the other problems and makes the whole situation worse. When I show someone that there is a way they can get out of feeling overwhelmed, that makes them feel better. Feeling better, in and of itself, helps to eliminate "being overwhelmed" as one of their problems. Now, they just have the existing problems to face.

I want to give you an analogy that I use often. The overwhelmed person feels like they are in a pitch-black cave with no light. It is scary and disturbing. The person tries to get up but hits his head on the ceiling of the cave. He goes to his right but touches a wall that is slimy. He goes to his left and hits something sharp and painful. Forward is a solid rock. Backwards is icy. The person has tried different ways to get out but is met with insurmountable obstacles. This person gets overwhelmed and sits down, resigned to never getting out, to having to stay the rest of his life in a dark, cold cave. If you've been overwhelmed, this analogy hits home. If you have never felt overwhelmed, this example can serve to give you some empathy.

In the context of this analogy, my job—and the reason you invited me into your home—is to provide even the tiniest of lights. The light can show you the way out of this cave. But you have to trust me. My regular patients have known me for years, but you are just getting to know me. If you are willing to let me show you some ways to stop feeling overwhelmed, read on.

To restate:

Being overwhelmed is a state when there are too many issues to attend to for the individual—or one unmanageably big one. It is based on fear and sadness. It is often mislabeled as depression. It can occur in other animals but is way more likely in humans because humans have so many more sources of stress.

The first treatment for *overwhelmed* is, as with other stressors, education. By understanding what is going on, it is easier to find a solution to the problem. After you have knowledge about what being overwhelmed constitutes, you have clearer ideas on how to address the problem.

There are many other solutions, and I will detail them in no particular order. One might be helpful for one person and another helpful for someone else. They can be used together or separately.

The traditional treatment is medication. There are many types of medication, but, in general, they all adjust some neurochemical in the brain to effect a change. The medications all have some benefit. Unfortunately, they also come with side effects. Your doctor can help you balance the benefits and side effects. Because there is no objective guide to follow, a lot of the medication use is really a trial. You try one medicine and see if the benefits outweigh the side effects for you. If that medication doesn't work or the side effects are intolerable, you try a different one. The trial period can go on until you find the medication or dosage that works best for you.

Since the majority of patients aren't chemically abnormal, I usually tell my patients that this medication is temporary. It is a quicker, convenient way to get a boost. It makes the patient feel better artificially. If someone feels better, a level-10 stressor might seem like an only level-8 stressor. That makes it easier to start to deal with the problem. The good news is that when the person no longer feels overwhelmed, they won't need to take the medication (unless they start feeling overwhelmed again). My patients find it reassuring to think they won't have to take this medication for the rest of their lives and that there are other things they can do to minimize or eliminate the need for medication.

You will need to talk to your own doctor for more details on what medication might be right for you.

Another area where you can make changes that can lower the feeling of being overwhelmed is with your perceptions. Your perceptions are your reality. It doesn't matter what is really going on: what is more relevant is your *perception* of what is going on. One way to deal with being overwhelmed is to try to look at things with a different perception or look at your life through a different lens.

The key to this perceptual change is the realization or admission that there *are* other ways to see any given situation. This is not easy for everyone. It might not be easy for anyone. You have to be willing to take off the perceptual goggles you have been using your entire life and try on a different pair. At first, this can be disorienting and distorting. Just as we learned in the section about worry, instead of focusing on the bad things that can happen, you can focus on the good things that can happen. Most perceptual goggles aren't equipped to look for the good. When I ask a worrier to tell me what good things could happen, there is usually a long pause followed by a very short answer. When I ask for a list of the bad things, it is immediate and lengthy. But a switch in goggles might make your life better—and that's worth the effort.

To make perceptual change easier to understand, I have been working on a new analogy. Its basis was given to me by my hypnosis teacher, Ron Klein. It is the idea of a map. I call it the "Adjustable Map." If I have a map of your hometown, it is not your hometown itself—it is a *representation* of your hometown.

Nonetheless, it makes it easier to get around. I can find your house or a local school by looking on the map. It gives me directions and distances, and shows the relationship between various entities in your town. But it is not your town.

There are many different types of map of your town. A map made by a cab driver, who needs to know the roads, will look different from a map used by an fisherman, who needs to know all the rivers and bays. Both of those maps will differ from the zoning-board map that predicts future growth *and* the map the utility man needs to locate a leaking drainage pipe. Each is a map of your town, but each also carries its own nuances, specific to its purpose.

In this same way, your brain/mind makes a map of your environment. It has the markings and landmarks that are important to you and your survival: Places to go and get services. Places to stay away from because they are dangerous. This map helps you navigate your environment. This map contains not just physical landmarks; it also includes people in your life. It has family members and friends. It identifies who is an ally and who is an enemy. Furthermore, it has a set of rules that act like a key and help you find your way around the map. It is not just a map of the present, either. It has a version of the past and a version of the future. The past is kept in chunks that need to be reassembled when called on. The future is in pencil and needs to be tested against the oncoming reality. This Adjustable Map is a tool. It is a tool we can use to help you find your way out of the black cave.

Let's look at your Adjustable Map. The first thing you notice is that it is *your* map. Someone else's map might show the same parameters, but it will look very different. That's the point.

Every person has a self-made, self-maintained, unique-to-them map. But the map is only a representation of your reality. It is not reality. You have been able to use your map to survive this far. That means it has been a successful map. It has not taken you off a cliff, drowned you, or let you be killed. You are still here, so it has been at least that successful. This map deserves your appreciation.

Your Adjustable Map, like every map, can be modified and tweaked to be more accurate or more efficient. You might need to add the new state highway, or maybe a Dunkin' Donuts has been converted to a Starbucks. Perhaps the speed limit was raised or an overpass added. Each day, there can be modifications. Sometimes you find the key is not as accurate as you would like. You might opt for distances in miles, not kilometers, or a map that is digital rather than on paper.

Maybe the past wasn't exactly as you saw it. You came to this new conclusion after attending a family reunion and talking to your uncle about the time you went fishing together. Maybe your future is not reflecting the changes you made in your 401(k) plan.

Your map is *your* map. You made it. It is a representation of your world, both physical and mental. It is adjustable as time goes on. It can be tweaked at your discretion to reflect changes in your environment and your outlook. You need to check your map against other maps to ensure it is as accurate as possible.

The critical strength of this analogy is your ability to change your map. You can make it bigger or smaller. More detailed or less detailed. Less focused on the past or more focused on the present or the future. You can make it the map of an fisherman or a delivery person. You can check with your surroundings and monitor its accuracy to see if the changes you make are helpful or not.

It is not easy to change your map—you have been using the same map for decades—but it is possible. By changing the map, you are not altering your core values. You're just changing their arrangement and the map key you use to get around. Don't be afraid to change your map. When you make a deliberate change, it is often for the best. Nevertheless, it can be changed back. Everyone could improve their sense of life if they just knew how. One of the ways is to change your map.

Most people have a fairly accurate map of their physical surroundings. It might need some detail shifted here or a detour added there. The most malleable part of the map is the key— sometimes called a *legend*—the tool that gives you the rules you need to interpret what is on the map. The key is where the most effective change can take place. If you look at your map of the world, there is a set of rules you use to navigate your environment. Frequently, you have been using the map for so long that it has been a good while since you even looked at the key.

I'm going to give you a few rules that many people have on their map, so you can see if you have them, too. These can be problematic rules. These rules can increase your stress. We'll work together to try to adjust them to reduce your stress.

The first rule: When I am with someone I love or with someone in a group I belong to, I tend to take on their stress as if it were mine. As a doctor, this is a common problem for me, as well as for my patients. Listening to your problems is what I do for a living. If I took on your stressors as my own, I wouldn't make it through the day without being overwhelmed. My patients are often overwhelmed not by their stress but by the stress of the people around them. I will sometimes ask a patient to tell me their stressors. Often, they list their mother's cancer, their brother's alcoholism, their daughter's difficulty at school, and the neighbor's money problems. When I repeat the question—tell me about *your* stress—I am often met with a pause. Patients have never separated *their* stress from the stress of those around them.

I can get rid of half your stress by modifying one thing in your key. Your stress maxes out at 10, but everyone else's stress is maxed out at 5. That may sound simple, but you'll find it is easier to say than to do. You have to be willing to listen to others' concerns and problems but not take them on as your own. You have to let others have their stressors and not make them yours.

I once had the honor of talking to the incoming interns in my residency. I gave them this advice, and I will give you the same advice. You need to build a wall around you. It has to be thick enough to protect you from others' stress and problems. And it has to be thin enough that you can still feel empathy.

I had to learn a lesson that I now teach patients: You can listen to others and offer advice and help, but you must be clear that someone else's problem is *their* problem—not yours. Even if their problem manages to leak through your wall, it can never exceed the level 5. Only your *own* problems get a max 10. Learning how to do this has kept me empathetic, allowing me to listen to thousands of patients and their families, while keeping me from becoming overwhelmed. I am here to do everything in my power to help and advise you. I will read books and articles, attend conferences, talk to my colleagues, listen with attention, call insurance companies or pharmacists to get what you need, and help you solve your problems. But it is *your* problem. I max out your problem at 5.

When your child comes home and complains about school, you can be empathetic and do everything in your power to help, but your child's problem must remain a 5 to you. Do not let it consume all of your energy, or you will quickly be overwhelmed. When your ailing grandmother is sick, you can help her in myriad ways, but her illness must be a 5 to you, not a 10.

There is a corollary to this: I can give you my best advice. I will work hard to make sure it is accurate and that you understand my suggestions. Whether you heed my advice, however, is up to you. I don't need to be offended if you don't take my advice.

I learned this from the book *Men Are from Mars, Women Are from Venus*. The author said men wear *Mr. Fix-it* hats. I disagree. I find just as many women wear *Ms. Fix-it* hats. Many times, the person complaining is just venting and doesn't want the problem fixed as much as they want to share the problem with you and have you listen. So, just listen. When you feel you might have a potential solution, then, by all means, share it—but don't be offended if they don't implement your proposed solution, no matter how smart it is.

You can work on your skills of persuasion or communication. You can find other new and practical solutions. But don't get mad when they come back the next day with the same problem. Just listen. You usually can't "fix" someone, so listening and offering advice without the expectation of compliance is the best thing you can do for most people. That approach keeps you from getting angry when the person doesn't follow your advice, which, in turn, saves you from ineffectual emotions and lets you be a better listener.

Now for the second corollary: If you make someone better off or happier because of their interaction with you today, you have accomplished a lot. You don't need to fix people. You *can't* fix people. You can only be their guide—and only if they let you. So, make your goal to help someone feel better. This is an achievable goal. If your goal is to make someone feel better, rather than to fix someone, you are less likely to suffer disappointment.

As a physician, my goal is to have my patient share at least one smile before leaving my office. There may have been tears, but, somewhere, there was a smile. At some point, the patient felt like someone listened to them and tried to understand and empathize. Someone gave them advice that didn't come with strings attached. Someone touched them, and they felt better because of it. I hope this book is giving you that same reassurance that I am doing everything I can to help you have less stress. Even so, it is your map and under your control. All I can do is advise and guide you to the best of my abilities.

"I can't do this anymore." I hear this statement all the time. It may mean *I can't handle this,* or *This is too much for me,* or *I'm exhausted,* or any of a number of variations. The bottom line is that *Life feels too hard. I don't want it to be this hard. I want it to go away. I want to quit. I want to feel happy.* Does any of this sound familiar?

It does! How can I help this?

Words and concepts are extremely powerful, yet they can be easily taken for granted. Saying *I can't do this anymore* makes your problem worse, not better. It does this in three ways. First, saying you can't do this anymore usually is not accurate. You are doing it now—you are still alive, and you usually can keep doing it. Saying you can't do it is like a sports team saying it can't win. It decreases the chances of winning and becomes a self-fulfilling prophecy. Second, this statement makes you feel out of control. You are doing something you have decided you *can't* do, which indicates someone or something is *making* you do it. This is not your choice. Your choice would be not to do it. Third, you feel like you are failing. Whatever task is in front of you, it is so hard that you just can't do it. You want to quit because it is so hard.

The inaccuracy, lack of control, and sense of failing make you feel bad, sad, mad. It sucks out your energy and spills it on the ground around you. It makes any overwhelming situation even worse. But remember that you are not alone. Many people feel this way. I hear this multiple times a day in my office.

Let's go back to Bridgette. She made a choice to divorce her husband. She knew it would put her on a more difficult road financially and physically. But thinking she that can't make a change feels even worse. She *is* doing it. Her kids are being taken care of. They have food and clothes, and they go to school. She needs to give herself credit for making it through a difficult time. Just recognizing that she is reinventing her life makes it seem less impossible and less overwhelming. Humans are amazing in what they can handle. The first thing I would tell Bridgette is "Congratulations for making it this far!" *Yeahhhh!*

Another tool to reduce feeling overwhelmed is a concept I had worked on but was crystallized by Tony Robbins. He uses the term *Transformational Vocabulary*. Essentially, this means *Words Matter*. Different words elicit different meanings and emotions. If I say *I hate you,* that makes you and me react differently than if I say *I don't like you right now.* Tony tells a story that, in hindsight, is funny but illustrative. He was in a meeting with his lawyer and his CEO. It came to light that a business associate was costing them hundreds of thousands of dollars. The CEO was red in the face and screaming that the associate was a bastard and that he was going to kill him. Tony was angry and upset; his heart rate was up, and he was breathing hard. He was going to teach the associate a lesson. The lawyer was sitting calmly and told the other two that he was peeved. He was going to have to figure out how to stop this business associate from taking advantage of him. The goal of all three men was the same: Stop the problem. But the three men's physical reactions, emotions, and vocabulary were all different. Which one would you be?

Tony decided that words mattered, and so he did an experiment. He would use different words. He was checking into a hotel late one night. His secretary had not booked the room ahead of time, so he was stuck, tired, and frustrated, getting himself checked in. The clerk could not have been slower if he had tried. Tony felt rage welling up inside of him, but he decided to try out his theory of Transformational Vocabulary. Instead of telling the clerk how incompetent he was and how he was keeping an exhausted man from his room, he said to the clerk, "I am starting to get peeved." The clerk looked at him in confusion. Tony repeated, "I am starting to get peeved." They looked at each other, and both began to laugh. Tony felt the anger drain out of him, and the clerk smiled and started working more efficiently. Tony got into his room, and, instead of trying to calm his anger, he was already relaxed and able to go to sleep.

Words matter. I have patients who tell me their pain is killing them. Or they think that getting an injection will be the worst pain they ever had. Their husband is a horrible ogre. Their child is a monster. Really? It's going to *kill you*? Your husband is an *ogre* or your child a *monster*? It is amazing how unaware people are of their vocabulary. I have to point out to patients what they just said and ask them if it's true. Then I suggest they try words that are less emotional. *My pain makes it hard to do things around the house* causes a different reaction than *My pain is killing me*. *My child is difficult* has a whole different ring to it than *My child is a monster*. *My husband is a wounded child from his own past* is way different from *He is an ogre*. These words matter. One way to feel less overwhelmed is to change your vocabulary. It will take some effort to become aware of the words you use—and then *more* effort to use different words—but it's worth the endeavor.

There is also another way to change. If the world appears as a bumpy road on your map, accept that the bumps are normal. Scott Peck wrote about this in his book *The Road Less Traveled*. It is not supposed to be smooth. It is bumpy 90 percent of the time. If you are lucky, it is smooth 10 percent of the time. Try not to see your road's bumps and detours and obstacles and ditches as abnormal. The fact that you are still here means that you have learned the life skills needed to navigate bumps and detours. Congratulate yourself for that. Instead of thinking the world is full of barriers, use your ingenuity (as you have done before) to get around or through them. By believing you can do that, you are more likely to make it. You are setting up success as a self-fulfilling prophecy. If you happen to hit stretches of your road that are smooth, be overjoyed at your luck.

What is taking place here is that you are regaining control. I had a patient who was overwhelmed with work. He was near retirement, and his boss was giving him the crappy assignments in an effort to get him to quit so he could be replaced with a younger, cheaper employee. My patient was miserable and said he couldn't do it anymore. Since he was near retirement, I asked him why he didn't just retire. He said he needed to work an extra year to get better benefits for the rest of his life. He did not see any choice in the matter. He was miserable and felt that he was not in control. All I did for this patient was point out that he actually was making it, that he had to keep at it for only one more year. He did have a choice, and he was making it: He could continue to work for a year so that he would have a better pension. He could quit at any time, although that option would come with a lower pension.

When he stopped to think about his choices, he came up with a reasonable solution. He had been a model employee who had saved vacation and sick time over his work years. He decided that, once a month for the next year, he would take a week off. He took back control. He thought positively, made it through the final year, and received the better pension. His road was bumpy, but he used his skills to navigate the final year of work to a more successful outcome. He stopped being overwhelmed. His positive ideas became a self-fulfilling prophecy.

Not everyone can find their solution as easily as that patient. But when you hear yourself saying *I can't do this anymore*, stop and think of the bumpy roads you have already traveled. Think of the choices you have—even if feels like two bad options, you still can choose. *Some* choice and control are better than *none*. Don't see things as barriers. Tap all your skills and those of your family, friends, and the professionals in your life to come up with a better way to get past the obstacles you face.

Another potential solution is found in the S curve we talked about earlier. In the S curve graph, you can see that, with one or two problems, you feel in control. The addition of a third problem steepens the curve, and you feel overwhelmed. Unfortunately, that feeling of being overwhelmed adds a fourth problem—making it all the more difficult to get yourself back under control.

But here's the good news. When you have too many problems, you don't have to solve them all at once to stop feeling overwhelmed.

The main objectives are:

1. Get rid of one problem.

2. Lower the intensity of all the problems.

3. Improve your ability to handle problems.

4. Don't lump your problems together.

If you look at the graph, three problems will make you overwhelmed. The fourth is the additional stress of *being* overwhelmed. So, it stands to reason that if you get rid of one problem, you actually are getting rid of two. Getting rid of one problem gets rid of that particular problem *and* the feeling of being overwhelmed. (Two for the price of one!) That brings you down to two problems, and two is manageable.

How do you get rid of a problem?

Solve one of the problems. That enables you to erase it. When people are overwhelmed, they tend to hold on to problems. You should try to counter that by solving a problem, enjoying that success, and moving on. Once a problem is solved, don't waste energy rehashing. Getting even *one* problem off your plate may be enough to lift you out of the feeling that you are overwhelmed. That, in turn, can free up energy to tackle the remaining problems. As an example, I have seen hypnosis in conjunction with NLP reframe a problem so that it is not a problem anymore. A patient who was biting her nails stopped after one session of NLP. She did not bite her nails again because she was able to reframe the problem and make it disappear. The mind has a lot of power that can be channeled to alleviate or change your perspective on a problem.

Ignore a problem. Typically, when I ask people about their problems, there is usually at least one problem they can do little about. Maybe they have to commute to work. Maybe their boss doesn't get it. You have to live with your in-laws. You have enough to deal with, so just let one of these problems go. Erase it from your list. You can't do much about it, it is draining valuable energy you need for more fixable problems, and it isn't life-threatening. So just banish it to a holding tank. You can always come back when you have more time and energy, when you're not overwhelmed. Don't waste money, time, emotions, or energy thinking about it, writing about it, or worrying about it. Put it in a corner, and forget about it for now. Focus your money, time, emotions, energy, thoughts, writing, or worrying on the problems you *can* do something about.

Lower the intensity of the problem. Medication falls in this category. An antidepressant can make every problem seem a little less intense. It might allow me to take three problems that are 10 in intensity and lower each to a 6. Now I have a total of 18, rather than 30. I have effectively lowered my whole S curve, and I don't feel so overwhelmed. There are a lot of strategies you can apply. Exercise, meditation, prayer, massage, for example, can lower the intensity of your problem. Pick one or two, and practice them. The more you use them, the better they will work. When I am overwhelmed, I play basketball or jog on a treadmill. My physical fatigue lowers the energy I can devote to stress over work-related issues. I can't focus on how big my problems are when I am using my available energy to make a layup or to keep from falling off the treadmill.

Improve your ability to handle problems. Counseling is one example. You can learn a lot about yourself and others from counseling. Counselors are teachers who can help you learn new ways to tackle problems. If you can't get to a counselor, there are books and blogs that you can use. This book can be one of them. These tools are more convenient and less expensive, but they aren't personal. One of my frustrations with a book is that I can't talk to you individually and ask about your personal map. I can't see your face to get feedback so that I know you are understanding me. I can only write in generic terms. Still, a book or a blog or a YouTube video can give you knowledge that can unlock a problem.

Share your problem with a professional or a friend. Don't be afraid to join a group. Maybe you don't have an answer, but someone else in the world might have the solution you need. Talk to people with similar problems, and put your heads together. Maybe someone you talk to will spark an idea that neither of you had thought about.

Don't lump. "Lumping" is something that almost everyone does from time to time, but it is counterproductive. Lumping means putting all your problems into one big heap. I have this one and that one and the other one and, oh, I almost forgot about the smaller one. I have to throw that one on top of the heap, too. You end up with a colossal mountain of problems—and guess what? It's overwhelming. How can you possibly solve this mountainous accumulation of problems and reduce the stress they cause? You can't even find the summit. It is too high to see. Fortunately, there is an antidote to lumping: Compartmentalization. Keep the problems separate.

How can I do that?

Good question. My friend Melissa gave me the answer. I want you to *think in terms of shoeboxes.*

Here's the picture: You walk into a bedroom, where you have 100 shoeboxes. When you open the door, there are 100 boxes, but everything is scattered about. A box is here, and the lid is there; the left shoe is over there, and the right shoe is over here; the crinkly paper that is used to pack shoes into shoeboxes just makes a total mess of this room. You can't even figure out where to begin to deal with the overwhelming chaos in front of you.

If you learn how to compartmentalize, you walk into a bedroom, and there are 100 boxes neatly stacked on shelves. The boxes and the lids are together; the left and right shoes are inside, with the crinkly paper wrapping them up. You are not overwhelmed even though there is the same number of boxes as before. You take one box down and open it up. You work with it; when you're finished, you put the lid back on and then move on to the next box. To feel less overwhelmed, I want you to *think in terms of shoeboxes.*

Sometimes, I find myself lumping. I literally have to stop myself and think *one problem at a time*—even if the problems are connected in some way. When I consider one problem at a time, it calms me down. Instead of inefficiently using my energy feeling overwhelmed, I can focus on the problem at hand. My chance of fixing the problem goes up as I narrow my focus to one problem.

I talk to my patients about lumping and compartmentalization. For some, the shoebox analogy is enough. But others need something more concrete. To help patients compartmentalize, I suggest writing. It takes more effort up front, but you have to do it only once. Use a loose-leaf notebook or a tablet of some kind. Take each problem, and assign it a separate page or a separate file. List the problem and why it is a problem. List any potential solutions that you can think of. Don't eliminate solutions at this point. Good ideas, crazy ideas, and even impossible ideas can all be written down. This is where creativity can play a role. Your problem has been around for a while, and it hasn't gone away, so you need something different. Letting your ideas flow, no matter how ridiculous, will stoke the creative fires. At worst, you'll smile at some of the outlandish solutions to a chronic, energy-sucking problem. Smiling is good.

After you have written down your problem, page by page, there are three steps you must complete. The first is to prioritize. One problem needs to be addressed today, and another can wait till next week. A third can be put in the closet for now. You get to decide the priorities and the time schedule. The second step is to make a to-do list. Too many people try to remember the things they need to do—and then forget them with the passage of time. By making a list, you don't waste valuable time and energy trying to remember what you're supposed to do. You can check off tasks as you complete them—and checking an item off the to-do list is a pleasure. It makes you feel good inside and reminds you of all the things you can accomplish. Third, show your written document to others. With a list, they don't need to guess at what's in your head. They can add solutions, tweak the problem, or even provide valuable insight that leads to a resolution.

The important thing about this exercise is to take *one problem at a time*. When you address the problems one at a time, it is rarely overwhelming. It is only when you lump all your problems together that they become a mountain so high that you can't even see the summit.

Bridgette sits down to write out her list of problems. Child care in one shoebox. Making money in another shoebox. Catching up on sleep in a third shoebox. And so on. When Bridgette takes the time to write out each problem, she has new understanding. She needs to get *one* job that pays her as much as the *two* jobs she currently has. She realizes her kids are old enough to do some chores around the house so she doesn't have to do it all. She also recognizes that her children are growing up and won't be around forever, so she'd better enjoy them while she can. Trace Adkins' song "You're Gonna Miss This" plays in her head, and she starts to cry. (Every time I hear that song, I cry, too, because my babies are now adults.) When Bridgette can't sleep at night, she looks at her problem list, checks what she has done and what she can do tomorrow, relaxes, and goes back to sleep. *One problem at a time.*

I want to briefly touch on the next level on the S curve after *Overwhelmed*, the level where someone is *Numb*. Again, this is a dangerous place. It is a place where someone is beyond being overwhelmed. The brain and body have a final safety valve, which, when it's engaged, shuts everything down. A person who has moved into this place can lose consciousness or might sit in a room and rock. This is the place where people can be suicidal, unable to see any way out. If you have an inkling that any person you know is past being overwhelmed and has given up, they need help right away. Get them to the hospital, to a doctor, to a psychologist, or to a counselor. This is as much of an emergency as a heart attack or a stroke. Don't delay. Don't let the person talk you out of getting them help. The numb person is not safe. Get them immediate help.

Because being overwhelmed comes from an accumulation of stress, the lessons of the previous chapters are also useful. Lowering or eliminating any stressor will help tamp down the feeling of being overwhelmed. Feel free to go back and reread previous chapters. If you've got a stressor I haven't addressed, be patient. My next book discusses six more stressors.

Now that you have read this chapter and understand being overwhelmed, let me know if you can think up any other techniques to reduce the feeling of being overwhelmed. Give me your suggestions on my website TheLessStressDoc.com.

LET'S RECAP

Definition of Overwhelmed

Being overwhelmed is a state in which there are either too many issues that require attention or one much-too-big one. It is based on fear and sadness. It is often mislabeled as "depression." It can occur in other animals but is way more likely in humans, because humans have so many more sources of stress.

Human Skill: problem solving, thinking, cooperative behavior
Side effect: fear, exhaustion, sadness, suicide
Tools:

- Change your Adjustable Map, change your reality.

- Limit other people's problems at a 5 max; your problems can be a 10 max.

- Give advice to others without expectations of compliance.

- Medication and counseling can help and should be needed only temporarily.

- Stop saying I can't do it anymore. That leads to negative consequences. Instead, realize you are making headway, and turn your success into a self-fulfilling prophecy.

- Use less-intense or less-emotional words. Transformational Vocabulary is effective.

- See life as a bumpy road with obstacles to overcome rather than impassable barriers.

- Consider hypnosis with NLP. Exercise, pray, meditate, read.

- Join a group that advocates for people who have similar problems.

- Think in terms of an S curve. The addition of just one problem can take you from being in control to feeling overwhelmed. That means eliminating just one problem can lower the intensity of all the problems.

- Improve your ability to handle problems by gaining knowledge and skills.

- Compartmentalize when you find yourself "lumping."

- Remember the shoeboxes.

- Take back control by seeing life as a series of choices even if they are difficult choices.

- Write down your problems. Make a prioritized to-do list, share it with others, check off the items as you accomplish the task, and revel in the success.

- If you identify someone who is beyond overwhelmed and is numb, rush the person to get help. NOW.

I hope this chapter brings you both a better understanding of what it means to be overwhelmed *and* possible solutions. Each chapter you complete is taking you closer to your Happy Place. Now, let's move on to the final chapter, which is also the most important one.

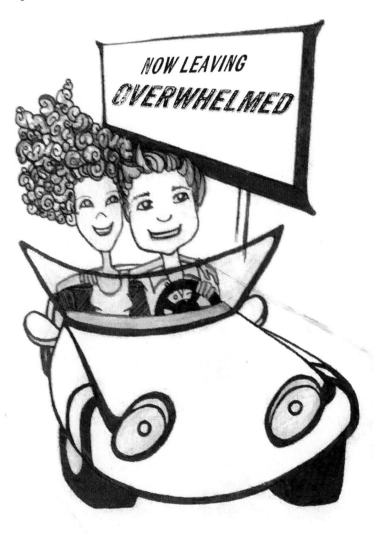

CHAPTER EIGHT

Change

Knowledge Is Not the Power.
Using the Knowledge Is Where the Power Comes From.

In this chapter, I will talk about how to make a change. I will show you the 5 steps to making a change. I will touch on issues that will keep you from changing and ways to negate or avoid them.

Making a change is not easy. But as I have emphasized throughout this book, knowing what you have to do to make a change is an essential part of eliminating stress. A deeper understanding of what you want to accomplish leads to better tools and more effective outcomes. Your life is marked by more stress and difficulties than you want. Sometimes you are so overwhelmed that you can't find contentment or happiness, or anticipate anything positive coming along. That's why you and I have come together. My goal is to help you achieve new outcomes that will endure for the rest of your life. I want you to look to your past, present, and future with a newfound insight that will enable you to live the life you envision in your dreams.

You have lived your whole life so far without making—or even knowing how to make—the changes recommended in this book. Don't be afraid to try them. Even when people are in a rut, it can be scary to think about breaking old habits. You can always find excuses not to change. You've no doubt heard them from others or even thought about them yourself. Here's one: *If I change jobs, I will be behind everyone else on the knowledge curve.* In the book *Range*, David Epstein, the author, shows that when people change jobs, it takes only a year or two to catch up with the majority of people in the new field. He reassures readers who are miserable in their jobs that change will feel better. Most people actually have multiple professions over their lifetime. Epstein encourages his readers to keep trying new opportunities until they find the job that fits best.

Here's another excuse: *What if people around me don't like the change?* This is a valid concern. When you change, the people around you must accommodate your change. There could be some pushback, especially if they didn't necessarily want you to change. But this is not insurmountable. You can alert these relationships that you are planning a change. You can try to make the change gradual. You can be patient while people get used to the new you. You may even find that you want (or need) to make new relationships.

There are whole books on how to make change. Jack Canfield's *The Success Principles*, Tony Robbins' *Awakening the Giant,* and James Clear's *Atomic Habits* are just a few. They are all worth reading because they give you some specific ways to make changes for the better and to maintain them.

I don't want you to read this book, make a New Year's resolution, and then be entrenched again in a rut full of stressors by

January 2nd. I want you to experience and enjoy new outcomes. I want you to be able to incorporate the information and insights you take away from this book into your daily life. It takes effort to make these changes, but the feedback that I have received from my patients has convinced me it is worth the time and energy. To help you on your journey, I have identified my own five steps that help make change easier.

What are the five steps?

Glad you asked. It just so happens I have spent some time investigating this issue.

1. Recognize there is a problem that requires a change.

2. Realize there are alternatives to your present attempt to solve the problem.

3. Figure out where you want to end up when your change is complete.

4. Act or think differently.

5. Repeat till it is automatic.

Let's examine these five steps in more detail.

Step One: Recognize there is a problem that requires change. This seems like it should be easy. *My job sucks. My spouse is my living hell. I have too many problems on my plate and can't get rid of any of them.* Sometimes it's easy to identify a problem. Other times, it takes more exploration. The exploration builds on two questions. *Does a problem exist?* and *Why is it a problem?*

Does a problem exist? Many of my patients drink alcohol. How many have a problem with alcohol? When does social drinking become problem drinking? When does it turn into alcoholism? These questions are not easy to ask or to answer. I have had to shed light on patients' use of alcohol too many times. Someone is getting a DUI, or their spouse is leaving them because of the drinking. The patient usually has come up with a defense. My spouse is crazy, and that is why I drink. The truth is that it is usually the other way around: *I drink, and that drives my spouse crazy.* Until you can see the problem, it is impossible to get a new outcome.

It often takes someone else's perspective to get clarity. That's what happened with my patient who came in with bronchitis. She smoked. She knew smoking was a problem and that it was probably playing a role in her having bronchitis. When we talked about the side effects of cigarettes, she revealed that she can't stop smoking, not even for a few hours. She told me she misses her sister, who lives in California. I asked why she doesn't visit her. She told me she can't stop smoking long enough for the plane ride. I returned the same information to her but with a new perspective—and that's when she finally got it. I told her one of the side effects of cigarettes is that she can't see her sister. She had never looked at it that way before, and it made a big impact on her.

Talking to someone about your problems opens the possibility that they will have insights that are useful to you. My daughter calls me frequently to run her thoughts and insights by me. She might already have an answer, but she wants my input. Is there a better answer? Does her answer make sense? This other person you select to speak with can be a family member, spouse, friend, therapist. It can be a group like AA or an internet group. Listen to the feedback you get from others around you. It will help you overcome what I call the "intention bias."

Intention bias occurs when you are assessing your own behavior. You filter your behavior through your intentions. If I see a mother punishing her child in the mall because the child ran away, the mother's intention might have been to keep their child safe and to teach the child not to do that again. She might paddle their butt to reinforce the message. But a stranger at the mall does not know what the mother's intentions are. All they see is an adult paddling a small child. It is important to seek other perspectives to avoid intention bias.

You've determined there is a problem, but you also need to understand *why* it's a problem. This takes some exploration—and you might need someone's help with it. Do you have a problem with your boss because he is a jerk? Or is it because he reminds you of your father, and you're mad at your father for the way he treated you when you were a child? On reflection, it might turn out your boss *is* a jerk. It is good to get as much insight into *why* something is a problem, including whether the cause is internal or external.

Let's assume you have the problem in focus now. Using Step 1, you realize your boss is a jerk because he yells at you in front of other employees, which embarrasses you. He criticizes you for little things and never gives you an "attaboy" when you do something beyond your normal scope of work. You worry he is going to fire you and then you won't be able to pay your bills. Your response has been to avoid your boss as much as possible, to put your head down and just do your work. You don't complain about anything at work. You just show up, do your job, and come home with a lump in your throat from all the worrying.

Step Two: To change, you need to find an alternative solution. You might have been in your situation for months or even years. Your response has kept you employed but at a significant cost. What other alternatives do you have? There are many possible changes you can make to get a different outcome. You could confront your boss. You could see him as a wounded child and, with some research, find out his wife is dying of cancer and that's why he is so irritable. You could look for a new job with a new boss. You could transfer to another part of the company. You could go to your boss's boss. You could give your boss an anonymous gift of *How to Win Friends and Influence People.* You could spend your nights learning a new skill and then change professions. You could quit and live in a tent in the woods.

The point I am making is that there are lots of alternatives. Some are good, some are painful. Some are easy; some are hard. Some are impossible. But you should let your mind explore every possibility before you reject it. Sometimes even crazy or outlandish ideas put you on a path that leads to other, more reasonable, solutions you hadn't considered. Once again, a relative, friend, counselor, or group might be of great help here. You aren't the first person to have an unreasonable boss. There are 7 billion people in the world. Someone out there certainly has had a similar experience and has come up with a solution that might apply to your situation.

It is important to remember that ***it is through choice that we gain control.*** We touched on this when we talked about regret. If you have no choice, you have no control. Having a choice, even if it is between two bad decisions, still gives you some control—and humans crave the feeling of control. You feel powerful when you get to choose your path. Many people overlook or ignore their choices, using claims like: "I have to do this. I have no choice." But you likely *do* have a choice. You likely *do* have a way to feel empowered and take back control of your life.

Alternatives can come in many forms. You could change your perception. It is your choice to see your boss as a jerk or a wounded child. You can change your map. Maybe being an engineer isn't working for you. What about switching careers to work on movie production? Maybe hypnosis, yoga, or mindfulness will help you. Maybe you need a new environment. Maybe a move is the right decision. Keep yourself open to all the alternatives at your disposal. Don't be too quick to eliminate possibilities. Empower yourself by seeing your life as a series of choices *you* get to make.

Step Three: Where do you want to be? I must admit, when I was writing this book, I focused on the first two steps and really didn't think about this question until much later. I spent a lot of time figuring out where stress was coming from and how to have less stress. But it wasn't until I heard my book consultant tell me that people don't care about the inner workings of the boat that is taking them across the lake—they want to know what is waiting for them on the other side. I realized I had to incorporate the Happy Place concept. The benefit from all of these stress-reduction techniques is not only less stress—it's to allow you to spend more time in your Happy Place. It is critical to know where you want to go. Otherwise, the roadmap is useless. Once you identify your destination, then you can start plotting your course to get there.

I spoke to a counselor who had an abusive husband. She was faced with a difficult situation, and she came up with three choices. She could try to make things better through counseling, learn to accommodate the abuse, or leave her marriage. Stress reduction was not helpful until she made a decision. Each path would require very different behaviors on the counselor's part. Until she decided what option she wanted, she was paralyzed. *Do I find a counselor or a lawyer? Do I call the police or find a safe place to hide in the house?* She needed to clarify what outcome she desired.

The counselor decided to leave. Once that decision was made, she mapped out a plan that took seven years to implement. But with a clear outcome in mind, she maintained her focus and eventually moved out of her home and into an apartment she had furnished. She had saved money to get her through the divorce process. She is now a happy woman. She was able to be patient and make decisions because she understood what she wanted to accomplish.

As a personal example, I decided I wanted to be a doctor when I was in junior high school. To this day, I don't know exactly why I decided that, but once the decision was made, the rest of my life came into clear focus. When faced with a decision about which high school or college course to take, for example, I opted for the one that would help me toward the goal of being a doctor. If something hindered my goal of being a doctor, I didn't do it. My friends who were undecided about their future didn't have that clarity. For them, selecting a course became an extremely difficult decision. They didn't know where they wanted to be.

Once you know where you want to go, the map and the highway you take are clearer—although not necessarily easier. Neither leaving your husband *nor* becoming a doctor is an easy task. While the journey may not be easier, the decision-making process is. When you are trying to change, it is critical that you know what you want to change and where you want to end up. Spend some time trying to figure out how being less stressed will impact your life and what you want to accomplish by having less stress.

Step Four: This is the act of change. To get a new outcome and leave the place you are in, you must act or think differently. You have spent some time identifying a problem, accepting the need for change, finding alternatives, and focusing on your outcome. This is the conclusive step, where you implement the change. There are two ways to do this. You can make a huge leap all at once, or you can make a gradual change.

There is an accountant who is a wonderful singer and has always wanted to be a professional entertainer. He makes a change—all at once. He quits his job as a CPA and goes all in on his new career. Making a leap all at once has both advantages and disadvantages. It fully commits you to a singular purpose. The CPA no longer has to try to be both an accountant and a singer. He is putting force behind his decision and taking away his safety net. There is no going back because he has quit his job as an accountant. He must do everything necessary to be successful at his new endeavor. Tony Robbins would say he is *taking massive action.*

Taking the leap quickly puts you in the place you want to be. It doesn't take patience to get there. The downside is that you and the people around you are quickly forced into significant change, and that can be disruptive. Ripping the Band-Aid off quickly rather than slowly sounds like a good, common-sense decision, but it hurts more in the short run. Taking away the safety net can also heighten the fear factor.

The other way to act or think differently is through gradual changes. In the book *Atomic Habits,* the author, James Clear, relies on the "1 percent rule." He uses the example of the British Cycling team. The team had never been a contender in cycling races. Then it got a new coach, who implemented the "1 percent rule." Every day, team members would try to improve by 1 percent. They improved their bikes, their conditioning, their gear, their mental preparation, their coaching. With this cumulative process of 1 percent changes, the British Cycling team won the Tour de France and multiple medals at the Olympics.

Gradual change has both advantages and disadvantages. Gradual changes are easier to implement. If you decide you are going to go on a diet, rather than become a vegan overnight, you can change a few things at a time. Stop eating meat first, and then add the other eating habits required of a vegan later. This has the advantage of giving you time to adjust to the new way of doing things and to incorporate the changes into your existing routine. It is also less jarring. Gradual change gives the people around you more time to adjust to your new preferences.

Let's imagine you want to start jogging. If you start out thinking you will run three miles a day, you will feel overwhelmed on your first day—you may even convince yourself that you don't have the time to begin the plan. Instead, start small. Make the decision to put on your running shoes. If you put on your running shoes, you are more likely to run. Decide to get on the treadmill for a minute. If you get on the treadmill for a minute, you are more likely to follow through on running longer. Small changes can add up over time and translate into big changes.

The downside is that gradual change requires more patience and diligence. You have to be committed to this new way of doing things. You have to be disciplined. You have to wait for results. You can more easily slip back to the old way of doing things.

But either way, to change requires that you do something different, that you overcome your fear, your opposition, and your self-doubt. With a thoroughly understood problem, a clear solution, and a dedicated goal, you will spend more time in your Happy Place.

Step Five: The last step is to make the change consistent. This is the hardest part. My patients will tell me it is easy to stop smoking. *Staying* stopped is what's hard. There is a good reason for this. It has to do with neuroanatomy. Thinking is difficult and time- and energy-consuming. Our brains were set up to operate *automatically*, so that we don't have to think. When I see a red light, I don't have to think about what to do. My brain has been trained to make me hit the brake and stop. There is a tract in the brain that connects a red light to hitting the brake. It is hardwired. Humans are amazing at making new tracts and connections. But the old tract never goes away. It can get rusty and overgrown, but it is still there. There is always the possibility of slipping back onto the old tract.

The key to lasting change is to make the new tract *automatic*. This occurs with repetition. The more use a tract gets, the more automatic the response becomes. If you decide your change is to jog more, the more often you jog, the more likely it will become an ingrained habit. Pick a routine, and follow it consistently. The more consistency, the more ingrained, the thicker the new neuronal tract, the more likely you are to follow the new tract, and the less likely you are to fall back onto the old tract.

After reading this book, you are going to decide whether you'll embrace realistic optimism. You have spent your life up to now being a pessimist. In deciding you are going to change, you will be more successful if you use realistic optimism every day. Eventually you won't have to struggle and think about realistic optimism. It will be automatic. Pessimism will be shunted to the back of your mind's closet.

Making this change will adjust one other important thing: your perception of yourself. Another word for expressing this is your *identity*. Before, your labeled portrait might have been "couch potato" or "pessimist." After your change, your labeled portrait will be "jogger" or "realistic optimist." This is an important shift. When you label yourself a jogger or a realistic optimist, guess what? You are more likely to behave like a jogger or realistic optimist. It is a positive feedback loop. You jog, you think of yourself as a jogger. What do joggers do? They jog. Doing it then makes it more likely you will continue to do it. And when others see you jogging consistently, eventually (sometimes quickly, sometimes slowly), they will change their perception of you, too. You now become their friend who jogs or their spouse who is a realistic optimist. Once again, this reinforces your positive feedback loop. It is all good.

One danger lurks behind change and consistency. It is deprivation. I take care of a lot of patients with stress-reducer loops (my term for addiction). One of biggest reasons they get derailed is because they feel deprived. The smoker who craves the cigarette that was given up. The alcoholic who wants just one drink. Deprivation takes energy to overcome. You need to block the old tract and focus on the new tract. What this requires will carry a cost. It might be the mental energy you'll need to say "No." It might be the money that will go to a counselor. It might be the physical exertion of doing something to avoid the feeling of deprivation. But what I have found is that, when you don't feel deprived, it takes no energy. I often challenge my smokers. I tell them to never eat mud again. Can you do that? They look at me like I'm crazy. They tell me, of course, they won't ever eat mud again. But here's the insight. Why is it so easy to never do something again? No one feels deprived that they can't eat mud. Giving up eating mud requires no energy because there is no deprivation.

How do I get rid of deprivation?

That question requires a complex answer. I will be addressing this topic in great detail in my upcoming book, *New Outcomes* (which offers a fresh way to look at addictions). For now, I can give you several tangible solutions.

First, don't look back. Whatever you are now is how you define yourself. Don't go back to an old definition. A patient of mine became a paraplegic after a car accident. He was deprived of the use of his legs. It took him some time, but, eventually, he came to the realization that he was never going to walk. He redefined himself. His labeled portrait was now "a paraplegic." It was no longer "a walker." Once he made that change, he wasn't deprived—he was just a person with paraplegia. He had removed the question of how he could go back to being a walker again. Once he did that, his feelings of being deprived left, and he became the most functional person with paraplegia that he could be.

Second, focus on the negatives of your old way. My patients who stopped smoking felt like they had given up a best friend. I understood their sentiment, but that feeling made it more difficult to stay away from cigarettes. Who wants to give up their best friend? What I told those patients was *to focus on getting rid of the risk of cancer and heart attack*. To eliminate the worry about whether the smell of cigarettes was offending someone (not to mention the real danger of secondhand smoke). By focusing on the negatives of the old habit, the feeling of deprivation was lessened, and staying on the new path became more enticing and easier to maintain.

Third, keep your attention on the positives of your change. By focusing on the positive outcomes of your change, you reinforce your decision to make the change in the first place. Why would you feel deprived if your life is better and you are spending more time in your Happy Place?

Deprivation is an important issue. It has undone many a person who has been trying to change.

Let me give you a personal example. When I was a young man, I weighed between 140 and 155 pounds. From medical school to my mid-50s, I weighed from 175 to 185. I have clothes that I wore for 20 years or more. But from my late 50s to my mid-60s, my weight went up to around 200 pounds. Despite gaining 30 to 40 pounds, I did not consider my weight a problem. But when the scale hit 200, I had to identify that there was a problem (Step 1). My pants were a struggle to button in the morning and almost impossible to button after lunch. I had difficulty bending over to put my shoes on. I did not like what I saw in the mirror after taking a shower.

Step 2 dictated that I find alternatives. I could exercise more. I bought a treadmill. That way, my exercise was not weather-dependent. I could eat less. I had eaten 2 bowls of cereal a day for breakfast for years. I began to skip breakfast and found I didn't miss it. Two meals a day was sufficient. I could buy new clothes. I found pants that had an elastic "fudge factor" built into the waist, as manufacturers found a way to add elastic to blue-jean fabric. I stopped weighing myself because my clothes told me in enough detail about where my weight was. I rationalized that I was getting older and my growth-hormone level and testosterone level were lower than they were when I was 20 years old. Finally, I enlisted my wife, and we found a plan called Optivia that included a diet that worked for us. We each lost 35 pounds. That was the alternative that worked. It was simple and maintainable.

Step 3 made me look at what my goal was. I did not want to be above 200 pounds. I wanted to look in the mirror and like what I saw. I was willing to attribute some of my weight gain to age—but not 200 pounds. I wanted my pants to fit. I wanted to tie my shoes easily. I wanted my struggles to enable others to deal with their own problems.

Step 4 meant taking action. I had to donate more jars of peanut butter and jelly that were in my cupboard than I care to tell you. I stopped going to local convenience stores to buy chocolate donuts and cookies while driving to work. I got on the treadmill at least 4 times a week. I had been playing basketball but added pickleball (a great game for older athletes), and dancing and singing. My wife and I followed the Optivia diet strictly and the weight loss was significant.

Then came Step 5. This is the hardest part. This is the part that takes commitment and energy. I had worked on this part multiple times and ended up back in my old habits. I had never let myself feel like a failure when I didn't achieve my outcome in the past. I knew that if I made some radical changes, like skipping breakfast, and some gradual changes, like going a little further and a little faster on the treadmill, that I could get the result that I wanted. As I am writing this book, I am at my goal weight. Optivia has changed my focus from weight loss to being healthy. I am in the process of laying down the tracts of new habits. I am finding alternatives to my old habits to lessen the feeling of deprivation. I don't dwell on my past, which is littered with less-successful outcomes. It is a work in progress. Sometimes, I'm at my goal, and sometimes, I'm working to get there, but, at least, I have clarity with the problem, the alternatives, the goal, the energy and commitment to change, and knowledge to make new tracts and avoid deprivation. Which makes the whole process easier.

My next goal is to improve my handwriting. (I am the poster child for poor penmanship and the definition of stereotypical doctor's indecipherable scribble.)

Now that you have read this chapter and understand change, let me know if you can think up any other techniques to make change easier. Give me your suggestions on my website The Less Stress Doc.com

TO RECAP:

There are five steps to change:

- Recognizing there is a problem and need for change.

- Finding alternative solutions.

- Identifying the goal of your change.

- Acting or thinking differently.

- Maintaining consistency to form an automatic tract and a change in your labeled portrait. Avoid deprivation.

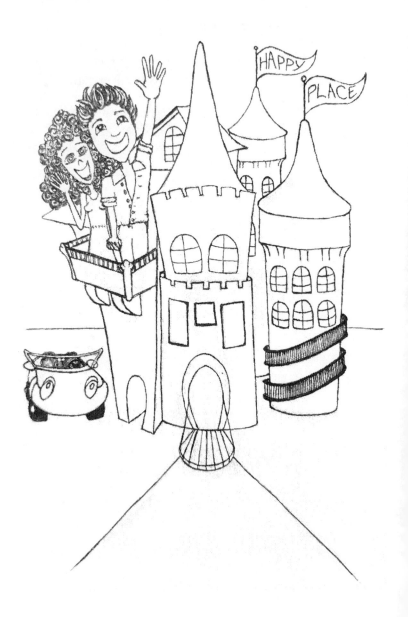

CHAPTER NINE

Destination: Happy Place

The map has you at your final destination, your Happy Place

Congratulations. You are at your Happy Place. I can give you two additional tools—a safe place and a competency tool. These can be used any time. I will encourage you to make these changes permanent. I will introduce you to some new spots on the map in my next book. I will direct you to my website to get further help.

Wow. *I have thrown a lot of information at you.* New concepts, new ways of thinking, new models, new terms, and new solutions. I hope what you have read makes sense to you. I work very hard to make sure you understand my insights, but I realize you now have a lot to process. I have had decades to get used to the findings on these pages, while you have had only the time it took to read this book.

I told you in the beginning that, as a doctor, I am used to seeing one patient at a time and getting immediate feedback on what the patient understands and, more importantly, what the patient *doesn't* understand. I can individualize my message and the solutions for the patients who come to my office. I don't have that ability with a book. But I want our relationship to be an interactive one, a collaborative one. That's why I have been working on how to get your feedback and individualize the message for you. I have come up with two ideas. (And I welcome your suggestions if you have others.)

One option is to present information on my website and create an interactive forum. The other option is to schedule a weekend retreat, where I can meet with you personally. Let me know if either or both of these makes sense and would interest you.

My teacher, Ron Klein, taught me an important lesson in one of his hypnosis classes. He told me that everyone already possesses all the tools they need to get a new outcome. That is such an empowering statement. What I have found is that you might need help finding those internal resources and building the confidence to use them to change.

Here are two tools I learned about in NLP class. They are called "anchors," but, really, they're tools. They're tools you already have. Once you are aware of them, you will find that they are always with you and that you can use them whenever the situation requires.

The first is the competency tool. I want you to reflect back on a time in your life when you felt supremely confident about your ability to do something. Maybe you're a teacher and you're supremely confident in your ability to teach a subject. One patient worked a printing press. He retired, but the company called him back because no one knew the press the way he did. One patient was supremely confident when he played "Call of Duty" on his PSP. Everyone has a time in their life when they felt competent. Maybe it was when learning to drive a car, cook a meal, or even tie your shoes. The more specific the incident, the more powerful it will be.

The teacher remembered when she had a student struggling with geometry. She used her teaching skills and recalled the look on the student's face on the day when he finally understood. She felt confident at that moment. My printing-press operator focused on the phone call from his boss asking him back. At that moment, he felt supremely confident in his abilities.

I want you to do the same. I want you to recapture the details of an incident that left you feeling absolutely confident. Mentally run over the experience, and remember the feeling that came with it. Think about it again to reinforce the recollection, which is your tool. Whenever you are feeling insecure or afraid, you can bring up this tool (which you always had) and again feel the rush of competence. This will help you get a positive outcome.

The second tool is the safety tool. This time, I want you to think of a time when you felt safe. Patients have talked about sitting in their father's lap or walking to the store holding their grandmother's hand. One patient felt safe when she was at a reunion, and all her family was there. Find your safe memory and recapture as much detail as you can. Make it as specific as you can. Don't just make it just a family reunion—make it the reunion in 2015 in North Carolina. Make it the memory of your grandmother holding your hand as you walked together to the Giant grocery store in Baltimore. You were 5 years old, wearing a spring jacket, and the sun was shining on you. It works. Go over the incident multiple times to cement the feeling. Then, whenever you are not feeling safe, you can bring up the image and the feeling of security that comes with it.

I have given these tools to many patients, and it is amazing how impactful they are. One patient chose a memory of his brother as his safety tool. Unfortunately, his brother had died. But the patient was able to retrieve a memory of his brother protecting him when he was being bullied in 5th grade. I watched the patient recall the incident, and his whole body posture changed. He was proud to have a powerful brother and felt honored that he was worthy of his brother's protection. He literally felt as if his brother was in the room that day. He now has the belief that his brother will protect him from heaven. He now has that tool/memory to use whenever he chooses. When he is not feeling safe, he can bring up that feeling of safety he felt with his brother, and it will help alleviate his fear. He always had the memory, but now he can bring it up on demand and feel better and less stressed. Better tools, better results.

I wrote this book because I wanted to help you. I genuinely hope you come away from reading it with knowledge that will make the rest of your life better. You already possess all the tools you need inside of you. You have the roadmap to find your way. You have the insights to get past the obstacles in your way. And you have the courage to make a change. I have given you a new way to look at things, so that you can alleviate your stressors—your worry, guilt, regret, boredom, low self-esteem, and the feeling of being overwhelmed. I applaud you for getting this far. Now take your roadmap, and begin the journey along the Happiness Highway and spend as much time living in your Happy Place.

I always thought knowledge is power. But after attending a Tony Robbins seminar, I had to adjust that thought. ***Using the knowledge you acquire is power.*** So, use the knowledge you have learned in this book, and go out and be a less-stressed person. Spend more time in your Happy Place. Enjoy all the amazing things that make up your life experience. Tell a friend about this book and watch them get happier, too.

Thank you again for reading this book. I am always honored that you have allowed me to touch your life. I know that you now have an expanded understanding of the sources of your stress and more efficient and effective ways to reduce your stress. You will now be able to spend more time in Your Happy Place. That is the place where you'll find contentment and peace, happiness, and the certainty that there is something better ahead. You will be filled with a sense of gratitude and of being fulfilled.

Appendix One

Strataspheres

Strataspheres is a tool that I have developed after reading multiple, eclectic books. It is a powerful tool that reshapes how you perceive your environment. I think it is groundbreaking because of the unique perspective it gives to the person using the tool. I think it helps answer questions that were unanswerable in the past such as how do you get a mind from a brain or what is love.

Developing Strataspheres was my original reason for starting on this journey. It led me to understanding where our mind comes from. But since I want to help people in a practical way, I realized that Strataspheres had shown me where most of human stress is coming from and so I shifted the focus of my work to alleviating stress. Understanding Strataspheres was not integral to you knowing how to reduce your stress just as knowing how an engine works is not integral to driving it or knowing how a cell phone works is not integral to calling your friend. Hence, I have relegated this topic to the appendix. That is not an indication of its importance to me, but rather it is a detail that is not mandatory for helping you.

What is Statasphenes?

Glad you asked. I actually struggle with what Strataspheres is. I concluded that Strataspheres is a tool. It is a tool that acts like a lens to the world around you. It changes your perception of what you see. It is a tool that can be used to reimage everything in your environment. It is a tool that can give you answers to questions that are unanswerable without it.

Another tool that we use already, as an example is the Venn diagram. In a Venn Diagram, (in its simplest form) there are two intersecting circles. You can then plug in the information you already have to gain a new insight. For example, one circle is yellow and the other circle is red. The place where the two circles intersect, where the colors overlap, is orange. This is a visual tool so while you could explain this to someone (like I just did), it is easier to understand if you show them the results of this tool. This tool gives you new insights into the information you have. Who thought yellow and red would make orange? This tool is used a lot in our world to gain new insight into existing information.

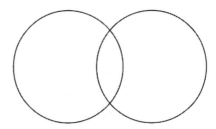

My tool is called Strataspheres. Think of Strataspheres as layered spheres. There is a core, then new layers are wrapped around the core. Here is a picture of what I am describing.

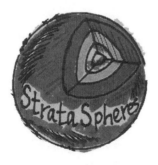

What makes Strat, spheres unique is how a new layer is added to the original structure—and what happens when a new layer is formed. The tool starts with a central core. Without this core, there is nothing. Inside the core there are elements. The elements can be anything. It could be letters or humans or brain cells. There are 2 important qualities to these elements. There is a quantity. There could be one human in the core or millions of brain cells in the core. Quantity is important.

The other quality is interaction. The elements need to be able to interact. It is the quantity and the interaction that leads to a threshold being crossed. When the threshold is crossed there is a new dependent layer added. This new dependent layer has new elements, and here is the key, the new elements have different properties than the elements in the core sphere. They are not greater than the sum, they are different than the sum.

The properties of a dependent sphere are not greater than the sum of its parts—The properties are totally different

These elements also have quantity and interaction and can combine to cross another threshold and another dependent layer is added.

The reverse process can also occur. If the quantity is reduced or the interactions are restricted, the threshold can be crossed and the new dependent layer disappears. The core sphere is essential for existence. The dependent spheres cannot exist without the core sphere, but the core sphere can exist without the dependent spheres. These are the basic rules of Stratospheres. This is the tool I have used to understand the brain/mind connection, complex emotions, the anatomy of a business etc. Some of these applications I will use in this book to help you understand how your brain works and hence where your stresses are coming from.

I think a couple of examples might make Stratospheres easier to understand. Let's say the core sphere is a single letter; we'll use the letter A. If the core sphere only has one letter not much happens. It just sits there. If I had 25 more letters but don't let them interact there is a little more diversity but, really, I just have a core with more individual letters. But here is the crux of Stratospheres: A new dependent layer will come into existence when there is a sufficient quantity of letters, and they interact. A threshold is crossed and a new dependent layer forms.

In this example, using the alphabet, the new dependent layer that emerges is words. This new sphere is essentially a unique group of letters stuck together. C-A-T or CAT. But here is the fascinating part, the properties of the words are *different* than the properties of the letters that form them. It is not that the whole is greater than the sum of its parts. **The whole is *different* than the sum of its parts**. What I can do with a word is totally distinct from what I can do with a letter.

In this simplistic example we're using, I can have letters and never have words. But I can't have words without letters. Letters are the core and words are the dependent sphere. I can add another layer when I reach a sufficient number of words and interactions. That takes me across another threshold, and

I now have a layer that is books. Books are made up of words, but they are also made up of letters. When was the last time you thought of a book as a bunch of letters? (Probably never). The term to describe the properties of the new sphere is emergent property. The properties emerge from the quantity and interaction of the inner sphere elements. The emergent properties are not necessarily predictable by looking at the properties of the inner sphere. It is also possible for a layer of the sphere to disappear. If the quantity or interactions are reduced, the process is reversed, and the dependent sphere will cease to exist.

Let me say it again. Strataspheres is a tool with a core sphere. A new sphere is added whenever there is a sufficient quantity of elements in the inner sphere and those elements interact to cross a threshold. The new sphere has emergent properties that make it different from the inner sphere. The core sphere is essential, the added spheres are dependent on the inner spheres for their existence. The dependent sphere can disappear if the threshold is crossed by decline in the quantity of elements or decline in interactions.

Here's another example. I am a single human. I am in the center sphere. If I was all alone there would be a significant limit on what I could do. Sharing would not be possible. Who would I share with? It would not exist. If I add other humans but they are spread around the Earth in a way I can't interact with them, sharing still doesn't exist. But if I put another human in the room with me a whole new layer forms. Whole new skills can emerge. Sharing can now exist because there is someone to share with. If the other human is the opposite sex, now we can have babies. With the addition of children comes a new layer called family. The properties or characteristics of family are different than a single human or even 2 adult humans. You can add another layer-group. This can be multiple families interacting. The characteristics of group are different than family, but they couldn't exist without families that are allowed to interact. A group sphere could go away if you are on a plane trip with your family and you crash on a desert island. You would lose the group sphere. But when you are rescued, the group sphere would return.

What does this have to do with my stress?

Everything.

Stratashpheres is the tool that leads to the explanation of how a human can form a mind from a bunch of neurons and neurochemicals. That leads to a separation of brain and mind but allows them to intimately interact.

Let's use Strataspheres to explore this brain/mind concept. In the core sphere we can put a brain. It has neurons and axons, blood vessels and connective tissue. It has spinal fluid and a protective covering. But guess what, so does a monkey brain or an ape brain. For that matter so does a rat brain. There are a lot of anatomical similarities between human and animal brains, which is why so much brain research is done on animals.

For thousands of years, scientists and philosophers have pondered the divergence between humans and animals. Although I don't profess to be smarter than any other scientist or philosopher, I believe Strataspheres offers a tool that might help explain the differences.

If the brain is in the core sphere, then Strataspheres suggests that with a sufficient number of neurons and the right connections, a threshold will be crossed, and a new sphere will develop with emergent properties. That is exactly what I think happened. A human brain isn't bigger than an ape brain or an elephant brain, but humans have the right kind of neurons and the right kinds of connections. When we crossed the threshold, the sphere we added was the mind.

The mind is the characteristic that separates humans from other animals. It is a small biological change. A few more neurons and a few more connections but, holy cow, the emergent properties that come into existence have taken humans—who are not that big, not that strong, don't have the best eyes or the biggest claws or the sharpest teeth—and transformed us into the dominant species on earth. Take a minute to soak in the enormity of that statement. We are the dominant species on earth because we have a few more neurons and connections that have led to a whole, never-before-existing sphere called the mind.

Using Strataspheres also implies there are humans who don't have a mind. As I wrote earlier in the book, newborns and patients with dementia have a brain but do not have a mind. Infants haven't crossed the threshold to a mind yet. Dementia patients have crossed back over the threshold of a mind. They are back to just having a brain.

Our mind is what separates us from other animals, so it is no wonder that most humans fear dementia more than they fear death and we always encourage our children to grow up.

Strataspheres can be used for other information as well. It can be used to re-envision business, politics, education, philosophy, etc. It can point to answers to questions like where did we come from? And where are we going? I have had decades to explore the implications of Strataspheres and it is exciting. But that is for another book.

Appendix Two

My unflattering professional journey

To begin, *picture yourself* in the waiting room of your high school principal's office. Your teacher turned you in for an infraction but you aren't sure what you did. You're sitting there sweating with fear, your fingers tremble, your heart is racing. You nervously watch the clock waiting for your meeting with the principal, your fate is in his hands. Your family will hear of this and become distressed. All you can think about is how bad the punishment will be and how fast can this be over with. The door to principal's office opens and your panic doubles.

Now fast forward two decades, you're an adult with a medical license and you are about to face your professional board. Your license is now in their hands. Your livelihood is on the line. All of your years of training can be taken away by a single vote of majority. Your ability to provide for your family and patients is hanging by a thread. This is the place I have found myself at for 2 decades.

I started my primary care private practice in a rural community to serve an traditionally underserved population. At the time, I began taking care of patients who were suffering from chronic pain. The medical community encouraged me to treat them aggresively. Chronic pain is huge problem in this country, and I was trying to do my part in alleviating their suffering. There were few pain specialists at the time, so I studied a lot and attended numerous conferences to make sure I was helping my patients and not hurting them. My board put out a letter to guide us, so I followed that letter and its guidelines.

Then the pendulum swung.

Now the medical community was punishing doctors for treating patients for pain. I went to court 3 times to defend myself. I had, as my expert, a physician who had practiced pain management for 20 years. The evidence showed all of my patients had pain, I followed the rules of my board in monitoring my patients, and most importantly, all my patients were doing better because of my care. No one was dying.

Each time the judge ruled against me their reasoning had nothing to do with the care of the patients. It was about hand-writing, charting, not liking my expert, or not agreeing with the standard of care I was following. I spent 18 months with a pain specialist and a psychiatrist that the board approved. At the end of the 18 months, both doctors wrote letters that stated I was practicing within the standard of care.

However the board was not satisfied with those recommendations. They created a new case along with four new doctors. These doctors reviewed the same charts that had been used to show I was practicing standard of care, and concluded that I was not practicing within the standard of care.

Obviously, using the standard of care as a benchmark can be difficult to define because it is a moving target that changes with the swing of the pendulum. At this point, the board wanted to take my medical license completely away. But, I negotiated a plea bargain that kept my medical license, at the cost of relinquishing my DEA license. This meant I could no longer treat chronic pain patients or treat patients with an opioid use disorder. Even though at the time, my treatment of patients with opioid use disorder had a 95% success rate. In the end, I was no longer allowed to care for those patients.

I didn't like what happened to me, but I felt worse for the patients. It became extremely difficult for them to find a doctor who was willing to treat their pain or opioid use disorder appropriately in this rural setting.

Soon after I relinquished my DEA license the CDC wrote a letter to all doctors. To put it in simple terms, the letter told doctors not to reduce patient's pain medications involuntarily. This was because more patients were dying and suffering because their pain was not adequately controlled. After all this time, this letter confirmed the way I had treated my patients was appropriate and safe. I felt vindicated but it came too late to help my patients or me.

A second incident in my career occurred with a local hospital. Once again, the way medicine was practiced was changing, and I was a pawn. Typically, I would see my patients in the hospital on my morning rounds, but then the local hospital hired doctors to see these patients instead. At the time, this was a new arrangement. In essence, the hospital paid a corporate doctor to see my patients. Most primary care doctors had few patients in the hospital and they were glad to let the paid hospital doctors take over their patients care. However, because I took care of nursing home patients, I had many patients in the hospital. It made sense for me to provide continuity in their care. In addition to continuity, it also kept me engaged in the local physician community. Unfortunately, every time I saw a patient the hospital lost money, so they decided my privilages to practice at the hospital needed to be rescinded. Once again, a case was created and they declared I did not properly care for a patient. The Chairman of the Family Practice at University of Maryland testified on my behalf, but it was for naught. In the end the hospital got its way, and I was forced to leave the hospital.

During all of these events, there was a significant amount of stress for me, my family and my patients. It was an extremely difficult time. I felt like I had a 55 gallon of stress, the concepts of this book were truly put to the test during this time. Honestly, I was only able to navigate this tumultuous time because of the tools that are in this book. If I didn't have the tools from this book, my family and patients would not have made it through those times.

During this time, I learned an incredible amount about stress and its effects on the mind, body, and relationships. From these situations, I am a better and more empathetic doctor. Now, when my patients tell me about their stress I can nod in acknowledgement and say with conviction, "I know where you are coming from. I have been there myself."

I have always had my patient's best interest in mind. I was willing to go to bat for what I thought my patients needed, and the people that know me know how much I was truly willing to do for my patients. Through all this time, my patients have honored me by calling me their physician. I did everything I could to care for them, and to deserve their honor and respect. I hope you will see past the pendulum shifts in medicine and understand that I have always cared for my patients to the best of my abilities. Your health and well-being will always be my priority and I will work every day to fulfill that mandate.

Bibliography

Morris, Desmond. *The Naked Ape*. Vintage, 2005.

Sapolsky, Robert M. *Why Zebras Don't Get Ulcers: The Acclaimed Guide to Stress, Stress-Related Diseases, and Coping*. Henry Holt and Co., 2004.

Canfield, Jack. *The Success Principles*. Mariner Books, 2015.

Zemeckis, Robert, director. *Cast Away*. 20th Century Fox, 2000.

Peterson, Jordan B., et al. *12 Rules for Life: An Antidote for Chaos*. Penguin, 2019.

Carbonell, David A. *The Worry Trick: How Your Brain Tricks You into Expecting the Worst and What You Can Do about It*. New Harbinger Publications, Inc., 2016.

Hoobyar, Tom, et al. *NLP: The Essential Guide to Neuro-Linguistic Programming*. HarperCollins, 2013.

Tutu, Desmond, et al. *The Book of Forgiving: The Fourfold Path for Healing Ourselves and Our World*. HarperOne, 2015.

Toffler, Alvin. *Future Shock*. Bantam Books, 1990.

Shadyac, Tom, director. *Liar Liar*. Imagine Entertainment, 1997.

Bigelow, Kathryn, director. *The Hurt Locker*. Roadshow, 2008.

Schaffner, Franklin J, director. *Papillon*. Allied Artists, 1973.

American Psychological Association. *Diagnostic and Statistical Manual of Mental Disorders Fifth Edition*. 2013.

Gray, John. *Men Are From Mars Women Are From Venus*. HarperCollins, 1992.

Peck, Scott. *The Road Less Traveled, Timeless Edition: A New Psychology of Love, Traditional Values and Spiritual Growth Paperback*. Touchstone, 2003.

Adkins, Trace. "You're Gonna Miss This." *Trace Adkins*, Capitol Records.

Epstein, David. *Range: Why Generalists Triumph in a Specialized World*. Riverhead Books, 2019.

Robbins, Tony. *Awaken The Giant Within*. Simon & Schuster, 1992.

Clear, James. *Atomic Habits*. Random House Business Books, 2015.

Frankl, Viktor E., et al. *Man's Search for Meaning*. Beacon Press, 2006. Andersen, Wayne

Scott. Dr. A's Habits of Health: *The Path to Permanent Weight Control, Optimal Health, and Wellbeing. Second ed., Habits of Health Press*, 2019.

About the Author

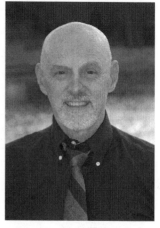

Dr Sprouse was born in 1956. He grew up in the Mid Atlantic region in a row house with his parents and 4 siblings. He started working as a newspaper boy at the age of 11, but decided by age 13 that he wanted to be a doctor to help people.

In high school he earned accolades as the captain of the wrestling team, scholastic athlete of the year and salutatorian of his class. He attended George Washington University for his Bachelor's Degree. He continued his studies at GWU for his medical school training where he graduated in the top 10% of his class.

Dr Sprouse set up his medical practice in an underserved area in the Eastern Shore of Maryland. During his years in practice, he has worked hard to be a relatable physician to his thousands of patients.

He has had a lot of stress throughout the years and has employed his own stress reducers. He sings karaoke, plays pick up basketball, travels, reads and loves to dress up for Halloween.

He has 2 adult children from his previous marriage and his current wife, Terri, has 2 children from her previous marriage. He has two grandchildren, so far.

This is his first time being a published author, but there are plans for many more books in the future. He is leading seminars on stress reduction. There is an online course for those that can't attend in person. He feels his unique and varied background and his skill for translating complex medical issues for his patients are the right combination to help people live a better life and spend more time in their Happy Place.

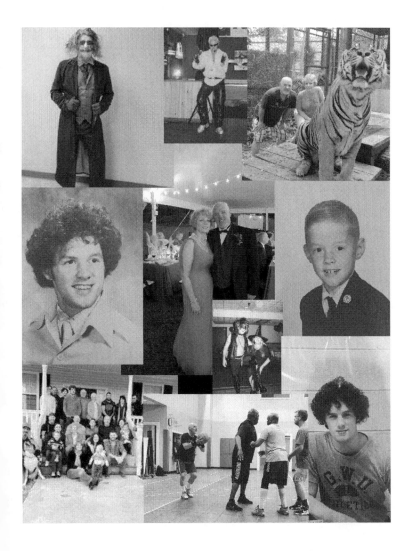